THE MOTHER'S VOICE

Strengthening Intimacy in Families

KATHY WEINGARTEN

The Guilford Press
NEW YORK   LONDON

The Guilford Press
A Division of Guilford Publications, Inc.
72 Spring Street, New York, NY 10012

Printed in the United States of America

This book is printed on acid-free paper

Last digit is print number 9 8 7 6 5 4 3 2 1

Library of Congress Cataloging-in-Publication Data

Weingarten, Kathy.
    The mother's voice : strengthening intimacy in families / Kathy
Weingarten.
        p.   cm.
    Includes bibliographical references.
    ISBN 1-57230-259-3 (pbk.)
    1. Mothers.   2. Communication in the family.   3. Family.
4. Intimacy (Psychology)   5. Fathers.   6. Sex role.   I. Title.
HQ759.W42   1997
306.87—dc21   97-24756
                                                            CIP

THE MOTHER'S VOICE

For Miranda and Ben
 and
to honor my mother,
Violet Weingarten

Preface to the Paperback Edition

I am delighted to be writing a preface to the paperback edition of *The Mother's Voice*. I began writing the book in November, 1990, one month short of the two-year anniversary of my initial diagnosis with cancer. As I write this preface in December of 1996, it is eight years to the day of my diagnosis. Time still matters. Dates still have heft and significance. I am grateful to be well on this day of all days, and grateful that the paperback edition of the book will bring it to more readers. I care immensely about the ideas that I put forward in this book and they have served me well.

Shortly after *The Mother's Voice* found its original publisher in 1992, I was diagnosed with a local recurrence of breast cancer. I was part of a small group of women, approximately 8%, for whom radiation fails. I relied on every bit of the work that I had done to challenge dominant ideas, as recorded in this book, to survive the new phase of cancer treatment. As a mother, once again, I had to put my self-care above the needs of my children—not always but often. As a wife, I had to feel good about myself as a one-breasted woman in a culture that prizes breasts as a woman's crowning glory. As the mother of adolescents I had to believe that they would want to support me to help them make that happen.

I had found this new lump, like every other lump, myself. I called my surgeon, who saw me the same day. After examining me, he looked grim. "It's tiny," he said, "no bigger than a grain of sand. But it has to come out." The first of what turned out to be three surgeries was scheduled into his first open slot.

As we both had feared, the biopsy showed a malignancy. But my doctor was able to reassure me that, with surgery, my prognosis would not change from the first cancer diagnosis; I still had a better than even chance of surviving. Because the lump was so tiny, I asked to try a procedure to spare the breast, a hemimastectomy. My surgeon was willing to try, with the understanding that if the margins were not clear, or if the pathology showed other areas of malignancy, I would have a total mastectomy. This conversation, in which I was negotiating tissue, felt straightforward. It was the one I knew I had to have with my children that I dreaded.

Living with a mother who has had cancer is not easy. Ben, then 17 years old, and Miranda, then 14 years old, handled it in characteristic and different ways. Ben was immediately sympathetic and cautious. "We'll have to hope for the best. I'm sorry, Mom." End of discussion. Miranda was filled with rage and sorrow. "But I thought you were cured. Your doctor told you to tell me you were cured. What happened? What's going on here?" Her outrage and grief cycled back and forth, not just in the first moments of my telling her, but for weeks.

I kept busy. I told a few people—family, close friends—but my appetite for talking about it was nonexistent. The surgeries felt more like all the routine monitoring that I manage on my own, without fanfare or support, than some new development.

I noticed immediately how much more in charge I felt than I had the first time. In the four and a half years since the initial diagnosis, I had learned a lot about breast cancer, about my style as a "patient," and about my doctors. I had relationships with all of my providers that felt sturdy and collaborative. In this crisis, I felt we were a team.

By coincidence, the day the pathology came back from the hemimastectomy, I was in my radiotherapist's office. He told me that the slides were inconclusive: Either there were cancer cells throughout the specimen, or there were dead cells. The team of pathologists had been unable to determine which was the case. Crushed and confused, I was nonetheless cheered by my husband, Hilary's, remarking that, with such a complicated finding, we at least knew that these were my slides! His comment made me feel validated and known to him.

Realizing that I now had to gear up for a mastectomy, I asked the radiologist to leave the office so that I could experience my feelings. I am proud of this. I broke the social convention and told my doctor that it was time for him to leave. By implication, I was also letting him know that, with him present, I would not be able to access or express my feelings. Of course, hospitals are not designed for people who have strong feelings—except, perhaps, for joy in maternity wards. I think that it would be a radical and desirable innovation for hospitals to provide soundproof rooms in which patients and family members could express their grief and rage. This would acknowledge the devastating effect that much of what happens in hospitals has on patients and their families.

A couple of hours after scheduling my mastectomy, I began to make plans for it. There were the logistics to arrange, but I also had a message to convey. I had asked my surgeon if he could make a vertical incision so that I could use the scar as the stem of a flower tattoo. He insisted that he could not perform the surgery that way and he lectured me about the dangers of a tattoo to my fragile, radiated skin. The conversation depressed me. I decided I would surprise him on the operating table with a tattoo on the breast he was about to remove. I spent several hours finding the right temporary tattoo, and after I did, I felt ready for the mastectomy. In fact, perversely, I relished my fantasy of his turning with his scrubbed hands to find the grotesque looking bulldog, with drool clinging to his fangs and a spiked club in his paw. I wanted the message to be, "I'm not giving this up with serenity."

I made an easy adjustment to being a one-breasted woman. Physically, I like the aesthetic of having an asymmetry on my body. I look part bird, part woman and I find this pleasing. Hilary doesn't find me less attractive, and I know that his sustained attentiveness has made a profound difference in my adjustment. Ben had little squeamishness and little interest either. He is supportive when I choose not to wear the prosthesis, whether or not he has friends around. Frankly, I'm not sure he notices.

Miranda had more work to do. At first, worried that her friends would find me "freaky," she was cautious about letting them see me without my prosthesis. Within a short period of time, however, after many long conversations about how cultural specifications of the perfect body are oppressive to persons, she became politicized herself. I would say that she is as staunch an advocate for the values I espouse in this book as anyone could be.

Clearly, the events associated with my cancer have affected the relationships in our family and have affected Ben's and Miranda's adolescence. They are more tuned in, more empathic, and more self-aware than many other children their age. They have participated in conversations about their mother's mortality which can only have been sobering for them, creating perspective at a very early age.

Yet they are joyful, open people. At this moment, with Ben nearly 21 and Miranda nearly 18, I can truly say that more often than not our interactions are intimate. The ideas I wrote about in *The Mother's Voice*, which seemed to be creating open, respectful, loving relationship, have continued to do so. I am convinced. And I am grateful.

My children's paths through adolescence, my journey with them and with the scores of families I have worked with during their children's adolescence, have made me wary of contemporary ideas about adolescence that describe it as a time of crisis and dissonance between parent and child. I am troubled by the adversarial metaphors that are used to describe this phase in the family life cycle and worried about the catastrophizing I read about young peoples' lives. My current work is devoted to offering alternative frameworks for thinking about adolescents in relation to their families that encourage the strengths and delights of this age. By providing other ways of thinking about this stage, I hope that families will be more likely to interpret adolescent behaviors in ways that promote pleasure and connection, not distance and despair.

Promoting connection remains my overriding goal. Fear of its loss does shadow my life. Yet, I am optimistic. In the last chapter of this book, I say that I would like to live to see the second millennium. It is close enough to hand that I can now say that I hope to see it. When I do, I will be looking at it with a vision shaped by the love and wisdom of many people, all of whom, I am sure, know who they are.

CONTENTS

ONE

Who Listens to Mothers' Stories?

> I think the key to . . . any sort of happiness isn't keeping your mouth shut but surfacing and experiencing every bit of life. To do so requires committing life to language, without which nothing recognizable as human can exist.
>
> —Nancy Mairs, *Carnal Acts*

I have been interested in mothers' stories for over forty years, ever since my mother told me one I could not understand. She was a marvelous storyteller, and I am sure she told me stories from the day I was born. I am sure she told me tales about cats and good fairies and taxi carrots that were ready to be put in my "garage" mouth. I am equally sure that she told me stories about her life. But I have no memory of any of her stories until the age of four, when my mother told me a story that made no sense to me. It was about her, but it was also about me. Though it is only a sentence, it is my first remembered maternal story.

My mother was employed full time as a newspaper reporter. I used to wait for her at the end of her day on my tricycle, at the entrance to our apartment building. I remember the sense of joy I felt when I spied her rounding our corner—not only would I get to be with her soon, but I also would get to pedal away from the doorway, out into the great big world of my city block, free and on my own in the space that was between the baby-sitter and my mother.

This world changed when I was four and my sister was eight. My mother quit her job, we moved to the suburbs, and my mother became, albeit briefly, what was then called a "housewife." The story she told me about why this happened was very brief. She said, "I wanted to be at home with you."

Some might call this sentence an explanation, not a story. But it was a story—the story she chose to share with me about why our lives had changed so dramatically. It was a story told to a young child who would presumably be thrilled that her mother wanted to spend more time with her. I was not thrilled. Hadn't she been at home with me before? Did this mean I must always be at home with her? What *did* she mean? I remember the confusion I felt; the sense that the tissue-thin layer that separated us had widened. The moment was riveting.

I do not think I am being fanciful to trace my interest in mothers' stories back so far, and to so short a story. Embedded in that impactful sentence was a longer and much more complicated tale—a tale about mothers, work, and family, a story about a mother and what she loved. My mother didn't tell me this longer story, because she could not. She told one assembled out of the elements available to her at that time—a story about the negative effects on children of maternal employment. She told me this story even though it contradicted her own experience, because she had neither language nor concepts to imagine her actual story without seeming to violate the well-being of her children. She was in an impossible bind. It has become my passion to help mothers tell the longer, more accurate versions of their stories. I want to help mothers, myself included, to untangle the binds we are in—to locate the words to create the ideas that will enable us to share the truths of our lives.

Story

Let me begin by clarifying what I mean by "story." We are all storymakers, making and remaking the stories of our own and others' lives. But we do so within certain constraints. Some stories in any culture become dominant, and it is then exceedingly difficult to tell tales that diverge. Cultures select some versions of stories to legitimate and others to deny, repress, trivialize, marginalize, and obscure. This happens in cultures at large, as in Western civilization, for example, and in small cultures, like medical wards and families.

I am using "story" to refer to the narrative form that a person gives to her thoughts, feelings, beliefs, and experiences. Stories can be very brief utterances, such as "Oh, my God," "Don't," "I love you," or intermediate in length, like the story a mother tells when she explains to her sixteen-year-old son why he must let her know where he is going to be when he goes out. And, of course, there are long stories, often renditions of one's life, that conform to the conventions of tragic, comic, dramatic, or romantic narratives.

According to the psychologist Jerome Bruner, narrative requires action, sequence, a sensitivity to what the culture deems acceptable, and, finally, a narrator's perspective or "voice." I think some mothers are so sensitive to the ways their feelings and experiences may *not* be acceptable to the culture that their ability to place their lives in story form is profoundly affected. Critically, then, for many mothers "voice" is affected too. A mother may silence or distort her voice in reaction to the contradictions she finds between what she believes (and others say) her experience should be, and what it simply is.

Two stories will illustrate my point. They are not really mothers' stories but, rather, those of the therapy hour in which the mother's story that was waiting to be told began to be elicited. That is what I do. I am a clinical psychologist who has been working as a family therapist for the last twenty years. I try to create an atmosphere in which the unsaid, and even the unknown, can be known and spoken. These two stories are examples of maternal stories that do not get told to children.

SUE'S STORY

Sue is the mother of a three-year-old daughter, Rebecca. She and her husband first came to see me when their firstborn and then only child, Sam, was diagnosed with a terminal illness at two years of age. I worked with them through that illness and death and then through the pregnancy and birth of Rebecca, at which time they took a break from therapy, because, as Sue put it, she could not feel merged with Rebecca and speak about her grief over Sam.

I have met with them individually and together for the last year. They come because Sue is chronically depressed and there are strains in the marriage. They have done their best to answer as simply and clearly as possible Rebecca's questions about Sam, whose pictures are displayed in the house. Sue feels she is always managing sadness; sometimes she can keep it at bay and sometimes she cannot. She and Bob are convinced that Sue's sadness is going to harm Rebecca. The other day Sue called for an extra meeting.

"Rebecca asked me where Sam was," she told me. "I told her he was in the cemetery. She kept on asking where in the cemetery. You know she's been there with us. So I finally told her, 'He's under a stone in the cemetery.' Later, I was worried that Rebecca wouldn't be able to handle this; that I'd done a terrible thing to tell her that Sam is under a stone. This morning she had another question. She said, 'Who put him under the stone?' I distracted her. There was a clown on the television, and I told her to look at him. I really don't know what to do."

Sue has a perspective on children that has been shaped by many experiences, not the least of which is the months she and her husband spent loving and caring for their increasingly vulnerable first child. Her belief in the vulnerability of children also comes from her childhood experiences with her own parents, who were not able to make Sue feel "undamaged" herself. In addition, she has selected—from the range of ideas about mothers in the cultures that have influenced her—the idea that mothers are ultimately responsible for the fate of their children. This belief manifests itself here in the idea that if Rebecca understood that her mother grieves for her firstborn child, that her mother's attention is not always with her, this would irreparably harm her. Consequently Sue, who is at home full time with Rebecca, silences herself as best she can. By this, I do not mean simply that she often falls out of speech, though this is also the case. Rather, I mean that she denies her feelings, splits them off where possible, responds to "meaningless" events in ways that are inexplicable to her, and suffers a debilitating depression that she and her husband find mysterious. "Why," they ask, "is Sue still having such a hard time?"

This anecdote is about a mother who conceals a central and vital part of who she is from her child, hoping that she can protect her child from the developmental interference she is sure would follow were she aware of her mother's pain. Sue restrains herself from sharing her experience with Rebecca. She has never said to her, "I'm sad." She has never allowed herself to cry in Rebecca's presence when Rebecca has asked a question about Sam.

I think Sue's depression can be understood as an accompaniment to the fundamental self-division she enacts daily. For in the process of protecting Rebecca from her story, she splits herself into the good mother who protects and the bad mother from whom her child must be protected.

CONNIE'S STORY

Connie's children are older. She has two teenage children who have both been hospitalized—Jane for running away and sexual promiscuity, and Brian for substance abuse, depression, and being suicidal. Connie has been divorced from the children's father since Jane was three years old, and remarried, to Jon, for ten years. The children call Jon their father.

I saw this family in consultation. Connie was the principal speaker and she seemed eager to answer any questions, but she seemed airbrushed from the events she had to relay. The outlines of the story were familiar. She had been abused by the children's father, her family had not believed her, and he had finally left

her with no money, two babies under two, and no idea of where
he was going. They have never seen him since. That was all in
the past.

Curious, I asked Connie if she had ever had a chance to tell
her story to anyone in detail.

"Oh, my God," she responded. "When I first met Jon, that's
all I did. He was the first person who listened to me and believed
me. I've spent hundreds of hours telling my story, to Jon, to
therapists—the kids' and mine. I truly believe it's behind me."

I then asked Jon, "Of all of you, who do you think knows best
what Connie went through?"

"Definitely, I do. Connie hasn't said much of anything to the
kids. We felt they were too young."

When she was asked, Connie said she was uncertain whether
or not she should tell her children more about her—and their—
early experience. She reminded me that no therapist had ever
suggested it would be useful.

An articulate, thoughtful, loving parent, she is desperate because her children are in so much pain. She is convinced that
the tumult of their early life as a family is responsible for their
problems today, but she is afraid to tell them what she remembers of those years for fear she might make matters worse.

I am convinced that Connie would have told her children her
story a long time ago if someone had challenged the idea that
she could make things worse for them. Embedded in the idea
that Connie could make things worse is a premise about maternal power that has a remarkable hold on her, and in our collective cultural imagination as well. Connie was utterly powerless
to influence her first husband's violence and abuse toward her,
or to arouse her family to come to her aid. Yet, ironically, it is
the story of these events, and her central powerlessness, that
now appears to be so powerful that it must be sanitized before
it can be aired.

Nobody has suggested to Connie that by *not* sharing her experience with her children, the children have been inadvertently
disconnected from a significant part of their mother, a part from

which they have much to learn. For what Connie would be sharing is not just events, but the meaning she has made of them, and the resolution she has struggled to achieve.

For both of these mothers, their stories about themselves have been constrained by their versions of the kinds of lives mothers are supposed to live. For Sue, mothers are supposed to be happy, not sad. Mothers are not supposed to be grieving the death of another child. Since she is sad as well as happy, she is violating what she believes her culture demands of mothers. She does not see herself as the madonna mother with a beatific smile that she feels she "should" be, for this image cannot contain the tear that runs down her cheek, touching the corner of her smile, filling her with a sharp sense of the fragility of life. She can find no cultural image that expresses her reality.

Nor can Connie. She, too, believes she is a mother "the wrong way." Though it is common knowledge now that women, often mothers, are abused by men in staggering numbers, it was not widely accepted when she was a victim of her husband's violence. She does not know how to speak to her children about something she believes she should have been able to avoid.

Voice

Sue's and Connie's maternal voices are silenced. Such silencing of maternal voice is not the choice of a solitary mother acting alone. It occurs in community, whereby some experiences are considered suitable and speakable and others are not. It is the rare mother who does not at some time have a story that violates a central idea of how she and her community think a "good" mother ought to be, feel, or behave. When this happens, with or without awareness, mothers are caught. They are caught between representing themselves accurately and representing themselves acceptably.

I know this dilemma well. I am a mother who has striven to be a good mother, avoiding those practices and feelings that violated my standards of what a good mother should be. At times,

I have squashed an insistent feeling—"What about me?," "I'm tired!," "I need . . ."—to satisfy a more relentless demand to put the children first. And when I have failed to put their needs ahead of my own, I have, indeed, slipped from voice to silence.

I have many examples of this, of which a dramatic one illustrates my point well. Several years ago, when my son, Ben, was ten and my daughter, Miranda, was seven, we flew home to Boston from Florida, where we had visited my father and his wife. I had last been to Florida eleven years before, when, pregnant with Ben, I had been visiting my mother, who was terminally ill with cancer. Every day of lying out in the sun with her was charged with the unspeakable and unknowable. Would she live to see this baby, now imperceptible within me? Would the love we shared pass through me to my child, forging connections of care after she was gone?

The more recent visit had been an intensely bittersweet few days, during which I returned with my children to the very spots where I had last been with my mother. We sat on the chaises where my mother and I had. I had been filled with longing, wishing, however hopelessly, that she could have lived.

On the return, preparing for takeoff, I was engrossed in myself, my own thoughts, my own grief. I had no interest in the children's arrangements—book bag here, stuffed animal there—and no patience either. I was mechanical, intervening only when essential. A few minutes into the flight, the pilot spoke to us. Due to a thunderstorm, he was going to have to make a sharp turn to the right to find safe passage north. Moments later the plane veered, and then dropped. There were gasps and screams, then absolute stillness, and finally the giddy sounds of people resuming life as usual—a more cheerful atmosphere than before, buoyed by the euphoria of relief.

I alone was inconsolable. My knees shook, my hands had turned to ice, I sat frozen in my seat, vigilant for every sound, sensitive to every motion. It was a nightmare flight; I was enclosed for four hours in profound panic.

It took me days to speak about what had happened, days before I retrieved the train of thoughts that had so panicked me that I had denied them on the spot. *I* could not have thought them. But I had. I believed that my thoughts revealed something truly shameful about me, some strand of being that lurked within, ready to undo my parental fitness. I thought I was confronting a self profoundly at odds with the self I desired to be— a shadow self, unreconstructed from the egotism of childhood, a nonmaternal, dangerous self.

Oh, my God, I am going to die, I had thought in those first few seconds of plunging. Only after I had reviewed and lost my own life had I turned, seconds later, to thoughts of Ben and Miranda perishing. In those lapsed seconds, with that sequence, I lost my faith in myself as a good mother. I violated my standards for being a mother. Of course I would not have talked to Ben and Miranda about this, but I did not want to risk sharing what I had learned with anyone else either. I silenced my voice.

Voice is a metaphor through which some people, especially women, it seems, express their sense of who they are, what they think, feel, know, believe, and care about. Voice is what we say, but also how we say it. In the best writing, authors have a distinctive voice. You can "hear" it.

Researching voice, I found a reference in a biography of Willa Cather, one of my favorite writers. A former music critic, Cather created an artful metaphor to describe her writing goal: "I was trying to sing a song that did not lie in my voice." She wanted to meld her song—her thoughts and feelings—with the voice that was her means of expressing it.

The metaphor of voice is useful because it simultaneously directs attention to the speaker and the listener. Cather seems to think of voice as something that can be found by turning inward, where she will discover her truest thoughts and feelings. Though I love Cather's image, the underlying conception seems wrong to me. I don't imagine that by turning inward I can discover my voice. Rather, I believe I must turn outward, to my community, to learn "what the traffic will bear." In effect, I am saying that voice is always social. Let me explain.

My mother was a writer, first a nonfiction writer and then a novelist, publishing four novels between the ages of fifty and

sixty-one, when she died. She wanted to be an old woman, because she believed that then, *then,* she would have "permission"
to be wise. A wise old lady. She died before she was old, and
before she had authorized herself to know, speak, or write all
that she might have. She died before she had entered that stage
of life in which she believed women have permission to be wise,
when women's voices are welcomed and can be heard.

I think that Cather is using the word "voice" the way someone
today might use the phrase "authentic voice." "Authentic voice"
suggests that a person can look within and discover what she
really thinks and feels. On the other hand, my mother had a
quite different notion. In her view, voice was not an individual's
achievement of self-knowledge, but a possibility that depended
on the kind of listeners that make up that person's community.
I think she believed that the issue was not whether you could
discover your authentic voice, but whether you could come to
know and share yourself without the crucial condition that you
felt well listened to and supported by others.

This shift from the idea of authentic voice to the idea that
voice depends on who listens to it has been central to me. It has
turned my attention away from voice itself to the contexts within
which voice is produced. It has made me deeply interested in
the conditions that are related to voice.

Writing is a form of voice, and there are conditions for my
own writing, this emergence into voice, for which I have a story.
It is the story of why I am writing this book now, not later, as I
had planned. It is the story of why I am writing a book about
myself, using my voice as a mother, daring to relate what I have
lived, when I had told myself repeatedly to wait until the children were grown.

It is a simple story: I could no longer wait. In the middle of
an average, innocuous, going-along-like-always day, I found a
lump in my breast, and it was cancer. This book is not the story
of the diagnosis or the treatment or the terror that came after,
though there is some of that in these pages. Instead, it is the
story of what I learned about myself as a mother that has allowed

me to write this book, upstairs in a study, while my children are still at home, in the kitchen without me, but not alone.

It is the story—my story—of how I learned about the hobbling ideas concerning mothers that constricted me and kept me in a vortex of contradictions, aswirl with "shoulds," "oughts," "dos," and "wants." It is the story of a better life now, one in which, more of the time, I do more of what I want, and believe that I am a good mother for it. This is a book about exploration, about a search for shards of beliefs and the bigger pattern to which they belong. It is the story of being a mother in late-twentieth-century America, having had a mother who did her mothering in the forties, fifties, and sixties, who was mothered herself from the First World War to the end of the Depression.

This book is also my answer to the question "As a mother, can I die my own way?" The question is an odd one, but unfortunately vital to me.

The day before my surgery, on December 4, 1988, a day when the lump in my breast was still just that, Hilary, my husband, the children, and I went to the ocean, about an hour away from our home. I felt the need to look into vastness. At the beach, the children and their friends romped; Miranda and Hilary actually went into the winter ocean for several minutes; and I paced the sand. It was unseasonably warm, maybe fifty degrees, a gray day with thick lowering clouds that skidded quickly by, backlit by the quirky light streaming through the higher layers of cloud. I thought, If I have cancer, and if I die, I will become a part of this, and this is not so bad. I will join the earth.

It was as if I were looking down on myself from a great height, attempting the kind of perspective one longs for when anticipating something dreadful and wanting to feel intact. The thought of joining the earth was momentarily comforting.

But then I had another thought, a dreadful one, eclipsing my comfort like a sudden bank of clouds: The same detachment that will keep me sane will be brutal for the kids. They'll want me to care all the way to the end, and I'll get through this only if I detach and pull away from them.

I felt pinned. I wanted to jump out of my skin, as if I could escape the conflict by abiding elsewhere. The conflict remained, my constant companion and, ultimately, the goad to write this book. In the months that followed, months of surgery, radiation, and chemotherapy, I thought often of what I needed for myself and what I believed my children needed from me. In my view our needs were often different: they required good cheer when I wanted a good cry; help with homework when I was desperate for a nap; a ride to school when I had a doctor's appointment. The conflict appeared in daily and ultimate ways.

I practiced imagining the unimaginable to see whether I could learn enough to make the unimaginable imaginable and manageable. I imagined my own dying, and thought I discovered there what I had discovered living: As a mother, I couldn't die in a way in which the central organizing bind of my life, which no perspective had released me from, would leave me. As a mother of young children, I couldn't die without its having a profound effect on them. In the scenes I imagined, there was always an intense conflict of interest between their wanting me to do everything to prolong my life and my wanting to do anything to cut short my suffering. I come honestly to represent the two points of view, for I have been a mother's child at her deathbed and I am a mother who can imagine her own.

Several months into treatment, I was driving with Miranda, then just turned ten, to pick up Ben at school. We had finished an errand.

"Mommy," she said, "have you decided whether you're going to be cremated or buried?"

I hesitated. I know my child well and I know the levels of response she expects and the hours of conversation that will follow, in time, from this comment. But we were doing errands, she was in her efficiency mode, and she wanted an answer. I'd have time to talk to her later.

"Yes," I said. "I'm pretty sure I want to be cremated."

"Oh," she said. "I want you to be buried, so I can have a place to come and visit you."

I was overwhelmed and I allowed a pause. Full of plans, she said, "What if we just cut off your foot, and scatter those ashes, and bury the rest of you?"

I was thrilled at my daughter's ingenious solution, and appalled. Just as I had known, I cannot die my way, for *my* self. I told her, "Many years from now, when only you and Ben and your partners and your children and your grandchildren are left to make the decision, I trust you to make a good one. Whatever you decide will be fine."

But it wasn't fine. Not really. I knew that I wanted something that was at odds with what she wanted, not just in this situation but in many others in our lives. I had been able to bear the tension of so many of these other conflicts of interest, but this one, with my resources vitally occupied elsewhere, sent me into a spin. I had to understand it. Why did I believe that there was a profound conflict between my needs as a mother and those of my children? Why did I find it so hard to speak about the conflict? Why did the conflict often show up anyway, in signs of frustration on my part, irritability, and impatience? Why didn't I speak to my daughter as honestly as she spoke to me?

These questions preoccupied me. What were the contexts within which I, the mother, felt unable to speak what I knew I felt, and she, the daughter, spoke, presumably freely, of her heart's desire? What context could so affect our relationship that I, who had encouraged Miranda to speak openly about her feelings, could censor my own? I watched and listened carefully, reading and thinking about this contradiction as much as I was able.

A year and a half later, at the beginning of her sixth-grade year, Miranda came home and reported the following story: "My teacher kept me after school today. I was talking and he looked at me and said, 'Amanda, stop talking.' So I turned to Megan and I said, 'I don't know who he's talking about.' So he looked at me again and said, 'Mandy, stop talking.' And I turned to the girls at my table and I said, 'This has nothing to do with me.' So he pointed at me and told me to stay after school. I did go up after school and, when all the kids were gone, he said, 'I was talking to you, and you talked when you should have been listening to me.' I said, 'My name is Miranda Worthen and I have been in your class for three and a half weeks, and until you know my name, I don't have to listen to you.' I was shaking when I said this to him."

Her story stunned me. I was proud, curious, and worried. I knew she had shown courage before, but I needed to know what her teacher had said next. "Nothing," she told me. I was flooded with questions. Did she speak this way because she knew her teacher could tolerate it? Had she known he would see her as assertive, not fresh? Did he hear her longing to be known as more primary than her criticism of him? Was he going to punish her in some subtle way? What did her teacher think the other teachers at this public school would find acceptable from a student? How did this conversation fit into the school environment?

The next day, I took Miranda to school and spoke for a few minutes to her teacher. He had heard her. Neither contrite nor angry, he felt she had made a reasonable point fairly. He had listened to her well.

This episode sealed my interest in thinking about how we listen to others. As a family therapist, I had always been interested in the context of people's actions, thoughts, and feelings, but I had thought about that context as consisting of relationships. I had assumed that if relationships were going well, people did share their thoughts and feelings. Now, this seemed inadequate. My relationships with my children were close, yet they didn't permit certain kinds of speaking. Miranda's relationship with her teacher was distant, yet she had spoken frankly to him. Perhaps, the broad category of "relationship" was insufficiently subtle to help one understand the reasons why some people speak up and others don't; why some people speak up some of the time but not always; why some people speak up some of the time about some issues but not others; and why some people do not speak at all about matters that are central to their lives.

I set out to understand these questions, not in the abstract, but in my own life. I wanted to understand what stopped me from asking my children to listen well to me. I wanted to understand whether what stopped me would stop them from doing so with others. I wanted to understand the context of the profound and disabling conflict I had felt since my treatment for cancer, a conflict that silenced and distorted my voice. In the months that followed I came to understand more vividly than ever before that, in addition to relationships, there is another context of voice: the ideas and values of the cultures within which we live.

TWO

~

The Good Plus the Bad Equals Mother

Dominant Ideas

People don't always speak what's on their mind. Sometimes they are so afraid of what the people around them will think of them that they can't allow themselves to figure out what they *do* think, or feel or desire. This is a way that relationships form a context for speaking.

But there is another context for speaking, more inclusive than relationships. In any culture, some ideas and values become more acceptable than others, and then become dominant, forcing alternative ideas and values to the margins, or underground. People whose ideas or feelings conflict with the dominant ones may feel awkward about expressing themselves, or may feel that they don't fit. They may be silent because they think they have nothing worth saying, or silent for fear that what they say will be dismissed or denigrated.

Unless people work very hard to avoid this, dominant ideas spring up in any group and in any culture. I have been interested in how small cultures—like radiation-treatment units and families—influence what we can know and say, as well as large cultures—like late-twentieth-century Euro-American culture.

What I Learned as a Cancer Patient

Ironically, perhaps, since I am an "expert" on families and not patienthood, it was during my cancer treatment that I began to appreciate how extensively one can be influenced by the prevailing norms of any group of which one is a member. Maybe because I was a foreigner in the land of cancer, I had a fuller perspective on the influence of dominant ideas and values in the context of that disease than I had in the context of mothering, with which I was all too familiar. However, the understanding I gained during my cancer treatment opened me to understanding my experience of mothering in a new way, for which I feel an abiding gratitude. I will summarize what I learned, for it did, truly, set the stage for what I have now understood about mothering.

During my cancer treatment I came to understand that the dominant ideas and values of a culture show up in the relationships we have with others, in the materials we read, and in the institutions with which we come into contact. Unbeknownst to me, I was flooded with normative ideas and values about cancer the moment I felt a lump in my breast, though of course I didn't know it at the time. A question like "Whom should I tell?" was supercharged with meaning. I was aware that my decisions were influenced by my desire to be "modern": I would be a person who talked openly of her cancer experiences, should the lump prove malignant, and I would not create a secret of my status. In this desire I was expressing and contributing to a current and, I believe, dominant way of thinking about cancer, one that reflects our growing understanding of the disease.

It seems that as we understand more about cancer, it becomes less terrifying to us, and we can imagine a friendly relationship to it, perhaps summarized best by the contemporary phrase "living well with cancer." It is a phrase that would have been literally unthinkable fifty years ago, when most people thought that cancer was always fatal, that its progression toward death was always horrific, and that treatments were aggressive attacks on a hidden enemy.

When cancer was considered an incurable disease whose course was invariably an "obscene" progression toward death, secrecy seemed the only moral response. So pervasive was this idea that medical textbooks advised physicians not to inform patients of their diagnosis; family members were enjoined to "protect" the ill member from the truth; hospital policy forbade staff to inform cancer patients of their condition; and, as enacted in 1966, the Freedom of Information Act cited "treatment for cancer" as the single exemption to the statute in which the law mandates disclosure.

Though I wanted to behave in accordance with this contemporary approach to cancer as "manageable," it hardly represented all of what I felt. To start, my mother had died of cancer and I had lived through her dying and death. The word "manageable" did not apply to the depth of pain, grief, frustration, and rage I had felt during and in the aftermath of her illness. In addition, as a child I had developed ideas about cancer that fit the prevailing ideas of the time—ideas about not only cancer but also its corollary, dying. Thus I entered my own cancer experience with a range of feelings and ideas, not all of which could be contained by, or were well represented by, the way of thinking about cancer I encountered at the hospital.

I vividly remember my first surgery, before the diagnosis had been established. Walking into the operating room I felt a palpable sympathy extended toward me. In my mind, I was linked to the nurses and the surgeons, yet in a few moments that might change.

While I was lying on the table, they talked to each other in a friendly, almost jocular fashion. Not offensively cheery. Not excluding me. They kept me posted as the operation progressed. I knew before they told me that they had seen the "lump." An eerie stillness filled the room; something common had become sacred. We entered ritual time—not just I, but they as well. It was awesome to be filled with their sorrow before any words had been exchanged. I felt cleanly dissected from the likes of them, the visible cells having cleaved a division between us.

Lying on that table, I suddenly cantilevered myself out of the operating room into a small rowboat without oars, preparing to cross over from the land of the people I loved to the land of cancer. Deeply absorbed in the picture of my transit, I must have registered my oarlessness and grasped the protest inherent in that image. I stopped the scene. I shouted to myself, "No! You don't have to go. You can ask your family to stay with you here."

But my "here" was not "manageable." It was—is—a place of confusion and contradictions; a place of seeking to understand for myself the emotional meaning that each moment, each step of the way, held for me. I would not, and so it seemed could not, feel what others suggested I should.

This resistance crystallized for me with my permanent tattoos, the little fragments of India ink that are pinched into your skin to direct the radiation treatments. I had been promised that my husband could be with me in the final moments of the procedure, for which I was sent to an institution neighboring the hospital where I got my care.

In a letter I sent the next day to my own radiotherapist, a person who had treated me with great respect, I wrote:

> My husband and I specifically requested that he be present with me while the markings were put on. The woman who brought me into the room told us that he could be there. In fact, at the end, someone approached me with the ink, and I asked whether my husband could be brought in. I was told "it won't hurt more than a pin prick." I then said, "I'm sure the pain is insignificant. I don't want him with me to support me because I may experience *pain*. It is the *meaning* of the markings that is significant, and I wish him to be present for that reason." She was clearly reluctant to delay her work and I capitulated. I was unable to put my need ahead of her need to conclude the task. I made a very bad decision for myself, and I take responsibility for it. I do wish the staff could understand that for some women, being permanently marked in the context of cancer treatment is not trivial. I

had wanted to counterpoise my own ritual of love and support to your ritual of marking me.

The radiotherapist's written response was swift and to the point. He said he was "concerned about our failure" and that he would do his best "to ensure that this situation will not occur again to another patient." Thus, I was mystified when I found myself literally unable to speak to him about my experience during the first few days of radiation at my hospital. Why couldn't I imagine that he would respond as sensitively to my spoken feelings as he had to the feelings I had expressed in my letter?

The radiation treatment suite at the hospital is attractive and comfortable. Procedures are explained clearly, and there is a support person available at all times. The men and women who strap and tape you to the table are kind, gentle, and inspire confidence. I always brought a friend. Why, then, I pondered, driving there and back, can I not stand this? Why do I feel so crazy here? Why are my thoughts racing, but not available? Why do I feel that I cannot speak?

Eight days went by. Simple days: Go to work. Leave work. Drive to hospital. Strip. Wait. Watch dying people get weaker every day. Walk to room and lie on cold, metal table. Lift arm. Be still. Be strapped. Be exceptionally still. Be left under a huge and noisy machine. Be alone. Alone. Be alone and be reminded that this is what cancer is all about. Cancer is about death, and death is alone, for a moment and forever. Be reprieved. Hear people come back into the room. Feel yourself unstrapped, untied. Walk back to your friend. Deal with your daze. Get dressed. Drive back to work. Work. Go home. Try to speak.

Simple. Easy. Only it wasn't, for me. Eight days went by, and the radiotherapist saw me in the hall. "It's not so bad, is it?" he asked politely.

I put my hand on his shoulder. I looked him in the eye. "It's worse," I said. "Much worse. Have you ever tried lying on that table, naked, alone in that room?"

"No, I haven't," he said. "Alone?"

"Alone."

"I couldn't possibly," he said. "That would be terrifying."

"That's my point. It is terrifying. To me."

Here in this good hospital, among the kindest of people trying to make a bum deal as good as it can get, I felt disqualified and invalidated. In prettying it up, in making the unbearable bearable, they left no room for my experience. Their solution to the problem of cancer—a problem of disease, sadness, and fear— produced more sadness, more fear. I could not speak. So different did I feel my voice to be, so foreign and out of place, that I might say their very thoughtfulness stopped my speaking.

Cotton balls applied gently in the throat can staunch sound as effectively as a fist. It is not only brutality that silences voice—though it does, profoundly. Benign conditions, reasonable standards, if they include no receptive listening, no space for difference, no room for alternative naming, can shut down and turn off voice.

Though I had no conceptual framework to explain what was happening to me then, I have gained one in retrospect to describe those first few days. All the careful arrangements—from the architecture of the bay windows overlooking the serene, never-used garden, to the cheerfulness of the attendants, to the ease of scheduling treatments—were mechanisms that conveyed the message that cancer was "manageable." These mechanisms were designed to express the dominant thinking about cancer to which the hospital and staff subscribed. They were designed to make me feel comfortable.

But I did not. Radiation hurt me. Seeing the deterioration of people sicker than I without a way of acknowledging it was disturbing, sad, and frustrating. I felt panic under the huge, noisy radiation machine, moving inexorably closer to me. I was profoundly at odds with the message embedded in the mechanisms, not because I disagreed with the content of the message itself, but because it excluded any other. I felt no room for other perceptions, feelings, ideas, or values.

Every day the attendants would say brightly, "And how are

you today?" and I could not respond. I was embarrassingly silent. Unable to figure out a way of commenting on the discrep-
ancy between what I was feeling and what I felt I was expected
to feel, I experienced confusion instead. It's not that I lacked
concepts or a vocabulary to express myself, but I couldn't make
use of these since there seemed to be no receptivity to hearing
what I *really* had to say.

Ideas become dominant not just because some words are used
more frequently than others, but because we use words to generate meanings among ourselves and these meanings become part
of our social world. So it was for me in radiation therapy. The
unit emphasized that their patients were "living well with cancer." How could I challenge that? If I did, would dissent be interpreted within the framework of the phrase? Would my distress
imply that I was not living *well* with cancer? What succinct
phrase could I use to counter the restrictive definition of that
one? Would anyone believe that "I'm terrified, unhappy, in pain,
and coping extremely well considering" was my equivalent
phrase?

Inadvertently, the radiation treatment unit made me feel powerless. The staff manifested their power in a critically important,
though infrequently discussed, way: through the appearance of
consensus. They had the means to produce a consensus of meaning—to *control* meaning—about radiation therapy and they did
so, rendering alternative meanings, and those who thought
them, marginal.

Temporarily, I also became frightened. What if they knew I
didn't agree with them? What if in response to their query "How
are you today?" I said, "Terrified"? Could my dissonant attitude
so disrupt the routine that a mistake could be made? I needed
them to treat me with the utmost precision. Did I need to conform to keep myself safe?

I began radiation therapy on March 6, 1989, three months
after the initial cancer diagnosis and surgeries and two months
after the start of my chemotherapy. I had survived those three
months emotionally by sharing my experience not only with

family and friends, but with my health-care providers as well. The beginning of radiation treatment was the first time I perceived such a profound separation between my experience and the experience others expected I would have.

In breast-cancer-treatment lore, "everybody" prefers radiation to chemotherapy. Initially, I did not. By the time my thirty-five treatments were over, the first tentative speaking I had begun in the corridor with my radiotherapist had become an ongoing conversation in which I felt his genuine interest and concern for me. Ironically, the rapidity with which I moved from silence to speech may have delayed my grasping the significance of what had happened to me. Perhaps if I had suffered silence longer, I would have been compelled to understand the mechanisms that generated my speechlessness sooner. As it was, it was nearly a year before I grasped that my experience in radiation was paradigmatic of the relationship between voice and dominant ideology in general. This understanding came only after I had spent another period in silence, this one longer and more profound— this time not in relation to my cancer treaters, but to my family.

A Dominant Idea about Mothers

Perhaps if I had not immediately performed a sleight of hand upon diagnosis, I would have made my descent into—and out of—silence sooner. It happened this way. I was driving back with Hilary from the appointment in which the surgeon had given us the details of my tumor and the menu of treatments and doctors available. I was on fast forward, planning, calculating. There were, now, staggering logistics to consider, choices to make. Yet I was stuck. A dodge loosened the jam. I said aloud, "I will have to make myself priority one, for if I don't, I won't survive to put the children first later. In order to be here for them, I have to take care of myself now." Thus I released myself to do what I had to do.

I also sidestepped having to question the premises in the psychological maneuver itself. Had I reflected, I might have noticed that I was operating with very specific ideas about what a mother should be like. These ideas intersected with ideas about cancer and produced a simple logic: I could believe that I was a good mother while putting my needs first. After all, my survival was uppermost for all of us. Napping, resting, not doing the endless trivial tasks a mother does, were my way of making myself available for the most aggressive treatment possible. It was only later, when I developed thoughts such as I might not finish chemotherapy, or I might choose to end my life if I were to learn I were terminally ill, that a system of ideas and values about motherhood that had been invisible to me became perceptible as I imagined violating them. It was as if I could be fully aware of these ideas only when I could no longer accept them.

The ideas about motherhood that no longer fit were ones I had taken for granted previously. These ideas and values, like the idea that "cancer is manageable," were played out in an intricate array of relationships—with my husband, friends, and children; the institutions I encountered as a mother (day-care facilities, schools, pediatrician's offices); materials I read (books, magazines, newspapers); and things I saw on television and in the movies. Everywhere I encountered messages about the criteria for being a good mother and the criteria for being a bad one. Clearly, in this time when I was exhausted from treatment, self-involved in the urgency of restoring my physical and emotional well-being, I was violating a central criterion of good motherhood: meet your children's needs first. Perhaps because I did not want to, perhaps because I could not, I became an outlaw to the code of mothering that I had embraced so eagerly when I became pregnant the first time. As an outlaw, having made myself newly strange to that which had been so familiar, I saw what I had never seen before. I saw the structure of ideas and values within which my mothering took place. What had been invisible to me became transparently visible, and I was terrified by that. I saw the dominant ideas that were controlling my life as a mother, and this knowledge did not make me happy.

"Good Mother"/"Bad Mother"

The central feature of the core idea about mothers that I perceived was its allocation of some thoughts, behaviors, and feelings into a "good mother" category and others into a "bad mother" category. Although my way of assigning thoughts, feelings, and actions to the two categories may have been idiosyncratic, the categories of "good mother"/"bad mother" that I used were ready-made. Thinking back, I realize that the categories were ones my mother used as well.

When I was eighteen, I was hospitalized for three weeks with an illness that had neurological symptoms. It took many days before the illness was definitively diagnosed. During that time I drew the erroneous conclusion from a spinal tap that I had a brain tumor, which meant to me that I would likely die. My mother visited every day, which made things infinitely better and also provided innumerable opportunities for me to vent my frustration, fear, and unhappiness on her.

After my discharge, someone suggested to my parents that it might be helpful for me to see a therapist to talk about what I had been through. My mother proposed this and I readily agreed. A few days before my appointment, she and I took a walk. It was late afternoon, and we walked through fields, up the crest of a small hill covered with tall grasses. "You don't want me to see Dr. Howard, do you?" I said.

"Not exactly," she replied. She was looking down at the ground, as if she needed to watch her step on this hill she had climbed hundreds of times. Her tone was resigned, and this time, like so many other times, I wondered what more she had to say, what more was going on for her. "I'm afraid you'll learn that I was a bad mother," she said slowly.

The late May afternoon was shining blues and yellows. We had set out together into the fields and hills to share the pleasure of the day with each other. I loved my mother and, at times, I hated her. I got along with her, was obnoxious to her, fought with her, adored her, all without a story line. Her comment was shocking to me.

I remember rushing to reassure her, speaking concretely to what she had said. "But you've been a wonderful mother. How could I possibly learn something that isn't true?"

Her words triggered a self-consciousness about relationships. But I didn't understand then what she meant. I knew only that she had said something crucially important and that it was not just about us. I knew that this was a moment to record permanently—that I would want to come back to it.

When I think now of my mother, I am amazed anew. She suspected that in therapy I would be subtly influenced to "discover" a particular story about my relationship with her, and yet this did not prevent her from encouraging me to go. This story, the story of the bad mother, was not only one of the most common story forms in the psychodynamically oriented therapy she knew about, but was a popular one as well. I appreciate now the irony of the good mother stoically accepting her transformation into a bad mother because it may be good for the daughter.

I remember being left with the puzzling question of how you could learn something about yourself that you didn't know or feel already. At that time, the idea of the unconscious mind seemed to provide the total answer. Now, I think that other concepts provide an answer as well.

I think my mother was aware, even if she couldn't name it as such, that there was an ideology of mothers, the central feature of which was the splitting of mothers into good and bad characteristics. She and I were caught up short by the rigidity of the dichotomization. It was as if the proverbial rug had been pulled out from underneath us. Our relationship—so rich, varied, complicated, and sturdy—was suddenly and simply either good or bad, one thing or another, implicated along with my mother in the polarization. In that moment, we both fell back on a ready-made idea about mothers: they are good or bad, one or the other. What they do, think, and feel is either good or bad. Simple. Too simple.

My mother was afraid I would assign her to the "bad mother" category, though she didn't specify what criteria she thought I would use. I have come to understand that mothers and others use all sorts of criteria to place a mother in the "good mother" or "bad mother" category. The reasons for an assignment vary substantially, but assignment itself seems common. I observe this all the time in my clinical practice.

A few months ago, a couple came in for an appointment and talked about a "devastating experience" the wife had had with their seven-year-old child. The mother had gone to pick up the child after a birthday party.

"I was on the stairs with her and I brushed against her, as light as a feather, and suddenly she screamed at the top of her lungs, 'I hate you, I hate you. You're bad.' I was absolutely shocked. I could feel myself freeze. I didn't hit her. I just looked at her and she looked at me and I said, 'We are leaving now.' When a mother and child we'd given a lift to got out of the car, I said to her, 'You have embarrassed me and humiliated me and I do not want to talk to you.'

"I could feel myself pull away from the mother cloth. I hated her back. I hated the way she made me feel. I felt I must be terrible to have produced a child who felt that way, but I just hated her. I wanted to withdraw. I could feel myself plummet. I know that it touched off a hurt in me that's very deep, that's from my childhood, and that is making me feel very, very depressed.

"Yesterday, she came over to me and apologized, and I put my arm around her and pulled her to me, but it's tentative. I told her that her apology helped. And then David spent most of the day with her, and we had a lovely family evening, as if things were starting to go back. But I know that something very deep has happened."

For the rest of the hour we discussed what the mother, and her husband, thought had happened. One part of our discussion focused on the daughter's saying "I hate you." The mother had felt exposed in public as a "bad" mother. In her community, she realized, mothers are supposed to be "good," their children are supposed to feel that their mothers are good mothers, and mothers and children are supposed to love each other. As we talked, it became clear that there were many ways, many situations in which she felt vulnerable to her child and to others viewing her as bad.

It is not surprising that she perceives the potential for judgment as a constant shadow. In her community—as represented by the institutions with which she deals, the texts she reads, and the relationships she has—maternal acts are frequently interpreted by others as good or bad. Even the most obvious of questions, such as "good or bad" for whom, may not get asked. Coincidentally, the day I met with this couple, the morning paper ran an article about a very pregnant movie star appearing nude on the cover of a national magazine. Experts were queried; essentially they were asked to code this mother-to-be's act as good or bad.

Shifts in Coding the Good versus the Bad Mother

Though coding maternal behavior as good or bad may be ubiquitous, what we code and how we code it has shifted dramatically over time. The feminist philosopher Elizabeth Badinter has concluded that mothers behave as the culture dictates. In her fascinating study of mothering practices in urban France from the seventeenth to the twentieth century, Badinter has been able to analyze that, for example, in eighteenth-century urban France, women of all classes did not organize their lives around the care of children, but, rather, around their husbands. A good mother did not breast-feed her children, as she might today, for this would interfere with her wifely role.

Ruth Block's analysis of colonial America supports the idea of cultural relativity. In colonial America, mothers did not devote themselves to their children. Instead, in the American context of hardship, the mother was a necessary member of the production team and she could not be spared to care for children, who were not seen as valuable until they, too, were old enough to contribute to the economic survival of the family and the colony.

The ideas about mothers that my mother, my client, and I appear to have shared are of recent vintage, as late as the nineteenth and early twentieth centuries. At that time, with the rise of capitalist states in which distinct roles for men and women came to be defined, mothers were seen as having responsibility for the home and the heart. Men were responsible for productive labor outside of the home, and women were responsible in the home for producing the citizens who would become the laborers needed to make the capitalist system work.

In the American context, the post-industrial revolution brought with it a need for skilled labor. Children became the hope of the economy and their training as productive citizens a critical task. The "discovery" of the child led to the "cult of motherhood." Images of mothers became polarized; mothers were either saintly, all-nurturing, and self-sacrificing, or cruel and ruthless. Though this history primarily fits white women of middle- and upper-class status, women of color and of lower social class were also affected by it.

Ironically, as children came to be more valued in this country, they came to be seen as too valuable to be left to mothers alone. The profession of the child-raising expert developed to assist mothers with their work. These experts, predominantly male physicians and psychologists, gave advice which itself shifted with the spirit of the times. A first phase was characterized by an approach based on the "principles of scientific management." John B. Watson, an earlier version of Dr. Benjamin Spock, recommended strict scheduling of babies in all areas and minimal affection. In "I Stand Here Ironing," Tillie Olsen's short story from the collection *Tell Me a Riddle,* the nameless mother remembers nursing her daughter according to the books: "I nursed all the children, but with her, with all the fierce rigidity of first motherhood, I did like the books *then said.* Though her cries battered me to trembling and my breasts ached with swollenness, I waited till the clock decreed" (italics added).

"Then said." Those two words convey the poignancy for mothers of doing what is "right" only to have right become "wrong." Dr. Spock's well-known book, published in 1946, captures the pendulum shift away from the theories of child development based on behaviorist principles to ones based on psychoanalysis. Himself a graduate of psychoanalysis, Spock's writing is emblematic of an era that placed greater value on the child's perspective as embodied by an adult—not necessarily greater value on children, per se—than on the mother's. Mothers were told to place affection at the heart of every interaction. Childcare was supposed to be fun. Mothers were to encourage the child's spontaneity and self-expression. The message to mothers was clear: The most important job in life is the rearing of healthy, well-adjusted children.

Thinking like a Child

I am suggesting that the core feature of much thinking about mothers is its reductive good/bad dichotomization. Though the content of what is considered good and bad varies over time and across place, and though different communities may evolve different expectations of good and bad mothers, categorization happens. However, it is important to consider whose perspective is encoded in the good mother/bad mother division. Nancy Chodorow, a psychoanalytically trained sociologist, and Susan Contratto, a psychologist, believe it is the child's perspective.

Chodorow and Contratto note that the adult assessment of mothers—by men and women, experts and nonexperts alike—curiously resembles infantile and early childhood thinking about mothers and is based on a "fantasy of the perfect mother." As Chodorow and Contratto point out, the fantasy of the perfect mother is partially produced by infantile fantasies that are themselves the outcome of being mothered exclusively by one woman. "If mothers have exclusive responsibility for infants who are totally dependent, then to the infant they are the source of all good and evil. . . . For the infant the mother is not someone with her own life, wants, needs, history, other social relationships, work. She is known only in her capacity as mother."

The fantasy of the perfect mother, which generates the good/bad split, obscures the mother's point of view. I think that my mother's conversation with me on the hill is a clear example of this. As an adult, she surely knew that perfectibility was not possible, and may also have believed that it wasn't desirable either. Yet the good/bad split left no space for her to locate her thoughts and feelings. These were pushed to the sidelines by her idea that she should be a perfect mother. I suspect that I, very much like my mother, took into adulthood the child's wish and fantasy that there could be, that I would be, that perfect mother.

Problems with the
Good Mother/Bad Mother Split

As I know from my own experience, and casual and clinical conversations as well, mothers vary considerably in the extent to which they are vulnerable to seeing themselves as bad mothers and capable of seeing themselves as good mothers. Some mothers seem mired in the perception of their "evilness," whereas others seem oblivious to any faults. Still others judge their every thought and deed, whereas others are satisfied to do the best they can. Despite a range of responses, a mother is made vulnerable by any thinking about mothers that contains a good/bad split. A mother is also made vulnerable when her thinking contains a good/bad split, because at those times she is likely to be thinking about herself from the perspective of the child she once was rather than the mother she now is.   Amen !

Thinking that expresses a good/bad split is likely, also, to transform partial descriptions into ones that overgeneralize. This creates two related difficulties. First, judgments about persons tend to be less nuanced and subtle than descriptions about what persons do, think, or feel. The result is that they are less helpful in guiding subsequent behavior. For instance, had my client's seven-year-old daughter shouted out, "Oh, Mommy, I hate it when you touch me like that, because it sends shivers down my arm and it gives me the creeps," my client might have been caught up short by her daughter's angry intensity, but she certainly would have known how to modify her behavior if she so chose.

The child's explosive "I hate you, I hate you. You're bad" contains no instruction for future interaction. It does, however, conform to a convention of thinking and speaking that is imaginable, even if painful. In fact, it is not just imaginable, it is common. Children don't spontaneously produce phrases like that; they are taught them by the communities they live in. That is, through interactions with family, friends, television, and books, they learn the kinds of expressions that conform to prevailing thought, including, especially, thinking about mothers. Children well past the age at which they are developmentally able to think specifically are not discouraged from making global judgments of their mothers. We, their caretakers, don't "hear" these remarks as fundamentally flawed. We may hear them as loving when enthusiastic—"Mommy, I love you. You're wonderful"—and angry or distressed when critical. But most of us are insensitive to the dilemmas produced by the categories themselves. Thus few of us challenge ourselves or others for using them.

After my treatment was over, I desperately needed to challenge my own self-assessment, but I could not. I was convinced that I had become a bad mother. Though capable of making fine distinctions about other people's behavior, I made only the grossest distinctions about my own. I was a bad mother, pure and simple. I had all the outward signs—irritability, impatience, and frequent anger—and, more important, the inward ones too. I didn't want to care for my children. I wanted to be alone, to rest, to do nothing for anybody else.

What's more, fundamentally I was terrified that I might die. The way I worked it out, if I died, I would be "abandoning" my children, an act so terrible it was punishable by death. That is, fearing that I might die led me to believe that I was such a bad mother I *should* die. Could I have invented such twisted logic on my own? I think the draconian punishment I imagined for myself took the idea of the bad mother to its ultimate, logical conclusion. It also fit with the habit of categorizing the total person rather than attending to specifics about her.

My thinking also fit with the second difficulty related to over-generalized descriptions like "good mother" and "bad mother." By judging myself a bad mother because I might die and thus abandon my children, I obliterated the context within which this might happen. Since mothers are judged good or bad, not actions, people infrequently focus on the context of maternal actions. Overgeneralization does not encourage the question "What is the context within which this mother's behavior makes sense?"

Thinking like a Mother

Children rarely ask qualifying questions about their mother's behavior. Oddly, many professionals often don't either. It is not uncommon for professional "experts" to develop hypotheses about, give advice to, and suggest interventions for mothers, all of which stem from their immersion in the child's point of view. It is particularly ironic when women therapists who are mothers speak or write in ways that are not informed by their own experience as mothers. I have sat for countless hours in case conferences where therapists who are mothers talk about client mothers as if there were no connection between their professional and personal worlds. When one does encounter crossover speech it often stands out as strikingly different.

Furthermore, such a professional, who suggests that her experience as a mother informs her professional expertise, often makes people uncomfortable. I understand that in this book, combining both personal and professional material, I am challenging conventional categories and, perhaps, perceptions. I hope to show that benefits may come from this.

Combining my roles may be a struggle, though. Recently an article appeared in my daily newspaper that made me realize how rare it is for mothers who are professionals to be invited to use the fullness of their life experience. The former director of the state Committee for Children and Youth was interviewed about whether she felt parents were entitled to know if a child had allegedly been sexually abused in a daycare facility in which their child was enrolled. The director said, "I'm sitting here wearing my professional hat and also wearing my parent hat." Asked by the male reporter whether when wearing her parent hat she would want to know about sexual abuse, she replied, "I would."

What is crucial is not the opinion itself, but that the two people were able to imagine benefit to the public in placing a maternal perspective alongside a professional one. In a modest but important way, this kind of exchange encourages others to value maternal thinking and to be open to ways of thinking about mothers produced by maternal thinking.

I want to encourage the legitimacy of maternal thinking and maternal voice, yet I am aware of how difficult it is for a mother to reveal herself in this way. The writer Tillie Olsen, speaking in 1962, stunned audiences with her observation that the voice of the mother is the most glaring absence in literature. Thirty years later, though we have countless works written by women, and women as daughters, the voice of the mother is still hard to find.

I am painfully aware of the difficulty of writing as a mother. There have been times when I felt unable to proceed with the writing of this book for fear that to do so, to show maternal thinking, to use maternal voice, would expose me either as a bad mother, a bad professional, or both. For if I write as a mother, I must share thoughts, feelings, and acts that have hitherto been excluded from the cultural dogma about mothers and mothering. Thus to write honestly involves the risk that I will be seen as bad precisely because what I have to say has been forced out of awareness, that is, marginalized.

Moreover, in writing as a mother, sharing my maternal thinking, I must expose not only myself, but also the children I love. While I can assume the risk of exposure for myself, what right do I have to ask them to share this risk with me? I cannot imagine any conditions under which a writing mother's child could give truly informed consent.

Nor could my clients, although there are ethical guidelines to follow in this case. As long as I protect their identity, I can write about their lives without revealing them. Yet, in writing about my own life, do I violate their right to learn about me in the context of their own uniquely evolving relationship to me?

No less disturbing, if I write about my experience, will I inadvertently marginalize someone else's? By writing a first-person narrative, am I breaking open the confining hold of one dominant set of ideas or merely displacing one version of a legitimated story—which at some level any story that is published has been—with another?

From Dominance to Diversity

The key to this concern about making a dominant story lies, I believe, in the word "displace." Any story that displaces another will replicate the problem of marginalizing other, different, tales. My hope is that my story can be placed alongside other maternal stories, creating multiple narratives expressed by multiple voices from multiple points of view. I am convinced that diversity, not dominance, provides the richest, and ultimately the most reliable, resource for us all.

I, however, can tell only my story, and I have chosen to do so from one perspective. When I write about my mother, I am trying to understand her experience as a mother, not mine as her daughter. When I write about my children, I do so from my point of view. And when I mention clients, I discuss those issues that resonate with my themes.

This book is my narrative in my voice. It is my hope that by presenting my story clearly and in detail, I will be giving the reader the opportunity that Gregory Bateson described as the bonus of depth perception. That is, if one understands what one eye sees and then puts this view alongside the view from the other eye, one can achieve perspective. I am counting on the reader to be the other "eye"/I.

My story, as it will unfold, is a story in which, oddly enough, cancer provided a perspective from which to observe myself as a mother in a new way. From the perspective of the newly strange, like a person who has traveled to a remote land and returns unfamiliar to the familiar, I took up the practice and thinking of mothering no longer immersed in it, but as if it were new to me. I saw that I was influenced by ideas and values that profoundly constrained my thinking, feeling, and behavior. I began to understand that I was not fully sharing myself with my children. I could see that a consequence of not sharing myself in planful, respectful, manageable ways was that pieces of feeling and thought escaped anyway, sometimes as unwelcome intrusions into my children's lives. Another mother, another mother's story, might be about the dilemmas of saying too much, with too much intensity, too frequently. And I hope that this book will create an opening for that story—any mother's story—to be heard.

Among other things, this book represents my effort to understand what impeded me from acting as collaboratively in my own family as I did in other settings. I wanted to understand why I was so willing to let my children express themselves, but so uncertain about how to express myself with them. Rejecting a model of authority and domination as a parental stance, I seemed at a loss as to how to apply the models of mutuality that were, and are, the core of my professional life.

In *The Chalice and the Blade,* Riane Eisler calls the shift from domination to partnership "a cultural transformation." I think that families can and must be part of this cultural transformation. This book is about just that. It is about challenging cultural beliefs that interfere with establishing mutuality in a family, told from one mother's point of view, in her mother's voice. The story, of course, starts and ends in mid-journey.

I am choosing to start at the stage in my journey when, returning to my life as a mother, I was newly strange to its routines. During that time, I identified ideas and feelings that constrained me from entering fully into partnerships. Among other things, this book is my effort at understanding the ideas—themes—that kept me from participating as fully with my family as I have tried in my professional practice to make room for others to do. Ideas or themes including responsibility, selflessness, wifely submission, power, violence, intimacy, and separation are ones I scrutinize, sharing my own experience, my clients', and the richness of other people's writings on these subjects.

I share a process of change—change made up of garden-variety, commonplace, daily happenings. I look at daily life up close, taking to heart Adrienne Rich's thought that women's work in their families is like a "million tiny stitches." If it seems that I dwell on trivial exchanges and insignificant matters, I agree: my focus is on the mundane. I believe that the ordinary is our nearest resource for change.

Always, my work is informed by the two decades of feminist analysis of motherhood, which, unfortunately, has not yet succeeded in rescuing mothers from the persistent dilemmas that make mothering so challenging. Mine is but another attempt in this effort. I am trying to illuminate my own life so that others, men and women alike, may see their lives illuminated too. I am hoping that my vision will draw forth multiple visions.

I think a lot about what would have to happen to allow multiple visions, multiple ideas to flourish. I see a field. This time it is not one I have walked on with my mother, but a field of fabric, a quilt. The quilt is of the type Elsa Barkley Brown describes African-American women crafting. Rather than valuing uniformity, she writes, they prefer variation. In their quilts, symmetry is achieved by diversity.

The image is useful and suggestive. It suggests that order can come without a center. I am trying to tell a story in this book that has no one center, and no periphery.

As a therapist, this kind of story is familiar to me. I work to help families operate in just this way, without one center and without a margin, but with multiple, shifting centers in which no one must hold, and any one can. In therapy, I help each person create a rich narrative, one that can be placed alongside others' narratives and understood. I am trying to write a narrative that can be placed alongside others—to write about myself as center, but in such a way that I make room for other centers.

~~~~~~~

THREE

Responsibility Gone Awry

But Anthony, I wanted to cry out, we have to give you
the illusion of safety, of order, or so we are told. . . . Our
lullabies are filled with assurances that nothing can harm
you, at least not until you spread your wings and take to
the sky. We are instructed, and it does seem right, to
place all sorts of boundaries around chaos for you—
rules, orderly rooms, assurances that, no, we will not die
until you are grown. . . .

—Jane Lazarre, *Worlds Beyond My Control*

Maternal Power

A mother of my acquaintance and I talk infrequently, but
we go quickly to the heart of the matter for us. She has three
grown children in their thirties; each but the middle child is
comfortably self-sufficient. My friend works long hours to be
economically independent herself. This second child has been
a heartache for his mother. Often pulled by him into areas
that feel like interpersonal jungles, my friend finds herself lost
in thickets of indecision, clueless, whereas in the rest of her
life she prides herself on knowing what she thinks and wants
to do.

With this child she has developed a voice she does not recognize as her own. It is a voice so tough, so firm that she finds herself actually mourning the sound of her other, loving, helpful, voice. With this son she has had to develop the belief that both voices are her. Finding the pitch of this harsher voice has been a challenge for her. Never having heard the voice she has needed, never having believed she would have to use it, she knows she has sometimes been strident when she could have been yielding. She knows, too, that sometimes she has been hostile when she could have been merely angry.

The steps along the way to discovering a tone she can bear have been marked with disconnection from her child. My friend tells me yet another painful episode in which she has been unable to think her way through a particular patch of confusion. Her child has asked her to rent a car for him, because he has a stubborn cough and thinks that taking public transportation to his job in the cold weather will be harmful.

"I gave him my old car," my friend says, "but he couldn't keep it on the road. He didn't take care of it; he let the insurance lapse. Now he is furious at me because I won't rent him a car. He tells me it will be my fault if he loses this job because he doesn't have a car to get there. I tell him, 'Honey, I wish I could do that for you, and obviously I don't want you to get sick, but I am not an inexhaustible supply source for you.'

"He told me that if I loved him and cared about him, I would do it. I get so confused. Should I rent a car for him? I gave him a car and he didn't take care of it. Should I do this? I know he doesn't feel well. I know he needs this job. He's probably thinking, There she goes again, always making rules and then sticking by them. Never any flexibility. But I don't think that's it. Am I wrong? Is he right? I thought I got past this long ago with him. I thought I had it figured out. I thought I understood what I needed to say to him, and here I am again. It's like a weight on my chest. I don't know what to do. I always know what to say with the other kids. Not that what I say is right, but I know what I want to say. With him, it's so confusing. I love him, but I cannot figure out what to say. Nothing seems right."

My friend experiences her confusion as unique to her. Hearing her, as I do, in the context of my search to understand the ideas about mothers and mothering that have caused me such distress, I recognize themes of my own. I recognize themes that my reading and thinking about mothers' lives—my own, my mother's, my clients'—have made salient for me.

I say to my friend, "It's as if no matter how old our children are, we still feel responsible for them. That is, if we are lucky enough to have maintained relationships with our children that are even reasonably close."

"Responsible, yes," she replies. "That's fine, some of the time. But why do I feel that he thinks my choice is to make everything work or else destroy his only chance? How does my being available as a resource get twisted around so that suddenly I'm either going to be a bitch or a saint? I don't want to be either."

My friend's belief that her son is going to see her as a bitch or as a saint, depending on whether she saves the day for him with a car, is an example of a dominant idea in action. My friend sees herself in a no-win situation. Frankly, she is as little interested in being seen as saintly as in being considered bitchy. Either way, she feels her position in her son's life is overinflated. She wants to be a resource, period. She doesn't want the power he is attributing to her, nor the responsibility that would accompany it. "I don't *have* the power," she has said, "and I don't want the responsibility."

Many mothers I have spoken to discover themselves in similar binds. Not only children have the infantile wish that a mother be all-powerful. The wish may come from adults as well, including, most insidiously, mothers themselves. No mother faced with the needs of her child doesn't sometimes wish that she were truly all-powerful, able to soothe, comfort, and "make it all better." Yet this natural wish is also a trap. For mothers are not omnipotent, and, depending on their time and place in the world, they may be more powerless than powerful.

Sara Ruddick has written eloquently about how difficult it is for a mother to keep her sense of her power in perspective, to separate out, if you will, what she and others may want from what is so. Any mother knows she has power in some situations. She is, after all, bigger than her child—at least for a time—and with size comes certain prerogatives, whether she uses them or not. For a while, she can also use words more effectively, so that she has resources to produce a consensus. She can say, "This is what there is for dinner. Take it or leave it" and go unchallenged. She can also say, "You may not cross the street" and teach a child sufficient self-restraint to keep him from harm in this circumstance. This kind of power is undeniable and is available to any mother whose child is capable of responding to her efforts of "preservative love, nurturance, and training."

Yet not all children are so capable. Some mothers painfully experience the limits of their power shortly after children are born. A baby who will not nurse. A child who cries inconsolably. A child who, the mother learns later, is autistic, blind, deaf, or retarded. But any child can present very real constraints on the mother's ability to feel powerful, because power is not a quality that inheres in a person, but is found in an interaction, in a situation.

Early theories of child development frequently missed the context of maternal "power." They were based on the child's perspective as told by and interpreted by adults trying to re-create and empathize with the experience of the child. These theories encoded what Chodorow and Contratto call "the myth of maternal omnipotence." Good mothers were powerful enough to create healthy children, and bad mothers were powerful enough to create dysfunctional ones. Neither notion has currency today with psychological researchers.

Embedded in these theories was an idea about mothers that reflected and simultaneously shaped prevailing thought about mothering; that is, mothers are responsible for the fate of their children. Yet this embedded premise, derived from the historical circumstances of postindustrialization and amplified by the child's, not the mother's, point of view, glossed over significant aspects of mothers' experiences and circumstances. Although delegated the task of raising competent children, few mothers feel assured that they will succeed.

In fact, there is a cruel irony for many mothers. They are held responsible for the fate of their children but do not have the means, the power, to provide the necessary resources to care for them. They cannot control, for example, whether their children live in safe neighborhoods, attend good schools, are abused by strangers, or are sent to wars. When the dominant ideology takes maternal responsibility as a fact, women are idealized when their children succeed and blamed when they do not.

Heartbreakingly, mothers internalize this blame themselves, even in circumstances in which their responsibility would seem farfetched indeed. I remember one session with a client in which she told me, half in jest and half seriously, about a recent episode with her son. Her three-year-old, angry at a male playmate, had walked over to her, pulled down his pants, and peed on the floor. "My first thought," she told me, "was, 'Oh, my God, I've ruined him already!' "

There are important variations in this way of thinking about maternal responsibility that, among other factors, depend on the extent to which people develop and sustain the illusion that mothers can be in control. For instance, as a group, African-American mothers and their children may have avoided the illusion of power and the disappointments attendant on the discovery of its limits. Although the acceptance of the mother's relative lack of power in the world may be a harsh reality, and the circumstances of racism and poverty that make this so may be heinous, children of African-American mothers may be less likely than children of middle-class white mothers to hold their mothers "personally responsible for not being able, through their individual efforts, to make basic changes in their lives or the lives of their children." African-American communities may not blame mothers as individuals for the problems their children experience, turning instead to socioeconomic and political factors for explanations. In addition, African-American communities recognize that their children may be better cared for if the responsibility is shared among biological and other mothers.

Voice and Maternal Responsibility

The ideas about mothers and mothering that are familiar to me are ones replete with idealization and blame, both of which depend on an acceptance of absolute maternal responsibility. Within this framework, what is unthinkable is the idea that the mother is not responsible. Autism and incest provide starkly powerful examples of the impact of ideas about absolute maternal responsibility. Autism is generally understood today as caused by defects in the neurophysiology of the brain. These biological defects produce profound and pervasive disturbances in the development of physical, social, emotional, and linguistic skills. Autistic children are unusual in many ways, as anyone who has taken care of or played with such a child knows. The child may repeat the same word over and over again and become enraged if anyone tries to stop him. Or he may become preoccupied with a single activity, like watching a record on a turntable, and refuse to do anything else for hours, or even days. Mothers used to be held solely responsible for aberrances of autistic children. These mothers were invariably found to be cold and rejecting. The children's oddities were believed to represent a defense against their hostile and unavailable mothers.

My mother's best friend's eldest child was autistic. Our families spent time together, but it is not the son I wish to remember; it is the mother. I knew that others thought she had done something wrong and that she, who did not think so, was astoundingly brave. My parents told me so. They admired Hattie without reserve, and I, not knowing why, watched her carefully to see what they thought so special. I missed, of course, the very thing I should have seen, for it was in her absolute assertion of her ordinary, good-enough mothering that her uniqueness lay.

Sue Miller, in her novel *Family Pictures,* vividly describes the repercussions for one mother and one family of blaming a mother for the autism of a child, a son born in 1948. The novel, written by a woman who knows the history of ideas about the etiology of autism, portrays the mother as consistently, though indirectly, resisting the definition of herself as blameworthy.

Trapped by a psychiatric perspective that "knew" the origins of autism were related to maternal deprivation, embodied in the novel by her psychiatrist husband, the mother nonetheless maintains a view of herself as nurturing and benign. Though unable to say she feels maligned by the prevailing psychiatric view, though silenced and out of voice, her actions in her family speak to her core conviction that she is not to blame and that she is not responsible for this child's, this family's, tragedy. At the same time, she cannot completely free herself from the tangles created by the insidious charges of maternal inadequacy that surround her. Her efforts to resist them, since they must be covert, sometimes boomerang and make her seem strange when she is merely driven to strange solutions.

Holding mothers responsible has affected the explanation for incest, as well. Until recently, mothers of daughters who were sexually abused by fathers were understood to be pathological, neglectful, and collusive in the incest itself. In fact, in the circumstances of father-daughter incest, mothers' responsibility was often deemed sufficient to exonerate fathers from responsibility. Professionals' blame of mothers of children who were abused prevented them from eliciting the actual experiences of those mothers. Having learned to appreciate the complex dynamics of coercion, violence, and secrecy that surround incestuous acts, we are now better able to hear mothers' experiences. When mothers were held responsible for incest, their ability to ally with the daughter in her recovery was compromised. Moreover, no one paid attention to the mother's grief. As a society, as we have developed concepts that hold men responsible for their acts of violence toward women and children, we have become able to see mothers differently. We can imagine a noncollusive mother, a mother, in fact, who suffers terribly when she learns— for she has not known—of her children's sexual abuse, whether by partners, relatives, friends, acquaintances, or strangers. Soon, I imagine, we will have novels and short stories that are written from the perspective of a narrator who will receive full sympathy from her readers if she tells about the victimization of her children. Soon, more nonfiction accounts will be brought forth by mothers who trust that they will not be held responsible.

A Tale of Responsibility Gone Awry

Some mothers faced with descriptions of themselves that do not fit their experience fall into silence, express themselves indirectly, or vent compulsively. Others lose their experience, becoming confused. Still others absorb the descriptions and take them on as truths. These then become ideas that *seem* to fit lived experience.

I am a mother who has absorbed the idea of maternal responsibility, colluding with a societal denial of my powerlessness to shape my children's destiny. Believing that if I were good I could take care of it all, I have unwittingly developed a matching maternal attitude, one of total responsibility. This attitude reveals a great deal about my circumstances, ones in which I could find ways to think myself in control even when, as in the case of my children's problems at birth, I patently was not. In fact, so ready have I been to adopt this attitude that I have raised the stakes: Not only have I accepted responsibility, but I have taken on "ultimate responsibility." Ultimate responsibility is to responsibility what omnipotence is to power. It is a response to socio-historical, familial, and personal factors, and it is a disaster.

I know. For months I was obsessed with the idea that I was "ruining" my children. This intrusive thought began in December 1988, when I received my cancer diagnosis through the intercession of an answering machine on whose otherwise empty tape I was told to call my surgeon immediately. Good news can wait; I knew I had cancer.

My nine- and twelve-year-old children were in the house; I had hot chocolate to make and car pools to drive. How do you tell your children that you have cancer when you only think you have? How do you explain that you may have to leave immediately and can't do any of what you and they have expected you

to do, when it is two days after a breast biopsy they know about
and about which they, too, are waiting to hear?

I called the doctor. He asked me to come to his office.

"My surgeon wants to see me, kids, so I have to go now. I'm
waiting for your dad to come and, meantime, I'll make the car-
pool arrangements so that you can get to your lesson, Miranda."

Ben says matter-of-factly, "You have cancer, Mom. I knew
you did."

Miranda throws herself on the floor and screams, "You have
cancer?"

Is this some bad joke? My kids have suddenly divvied up my
brain, and one is the optimistic side and the other the pessimis-
tic; one is believing, the other disbelieving.

"I don't know that I have cancer. I only know that the surgeon
wants to see me and that I promise to tell you the truth, whatever it is. I also know that, whatever it is, we have what it takes
to make it O.K. All of us. Together." And I flee to my neighbor.
I dump my news and the logistics of what should have been the
next two hours of my life. We hug each other; women, brave in
pain, connecting.

Now it is hours later. I do have cancer. My surgeon has been
more than kind; more than clear. Hilary and I have told the
children that I will be having an operation. Ben is clear, focused, reassuring.

"Many women get breast cancer," he tells me, "and if Nancy
Reagan can survive, you can too, Mom. Most women do now.
How does it feel to have Nancy Reagan's disease?" He attempts
a laugh. "I read about it in Newsweek before your surgery. I think
you have a ninety-nine percent chance. I know you're going to
be more cranky, which I don't like, but I can take more responsibility. I'm ready."

Miranda is wide-eyed and getting wider eyed. "I feel like
you're telling me I'm not going to be able to hug you after your
operation and I don't like that." She turns to her father, a physician, and is nearly still for a moment. Then she speaks slowly:
"Daddy, how can you stand being with people you know are
going to die?"

Hilary begins to answer. "Well, most of the people I see are old . . ."

Miranda flares at him. "I'm not asking you what you think. I'm asking what you feel. . . . I'm afraid that Mommy isn't going to be able to give me attention and you will be giving her attention and I won't get any."

"We'll get someone to take care of me, Miranda, so you can have Daddy take care of you," I reply, not thinking for an instant that this will solve her problem.

Hilary and I talk some more. We get up to make phone calls to our families, and Miranda jumps up on a chair and screams at us.

"You said this was a meeting to share feelings and all of you got to share all of your feelings and I didn't get to share all of mine and that makes me very angry."

We sit down. She has only one more sentence to say.

"Why am I the only one in this family that's scared?" she asks us.

The only one that's scared. The only one. Miranda, Miranda. The only one. It is hours later now, and I am in bed. I am trying to sort out my feelings, my life, my future, such as it may be. I am very lucid, as I will be for months.

"I will be fine," I tell Hilary, "as long as I can tell the kids I have done everything that was humanly possible to do."

But I cannot tell them this. I cannot say this, because some of what is humanly possible to do carries the risk of killing me later. I cannot promise them the one thing I believe they need more than anything else from me, the one thing I need. I cannot tell them that I will live, that I—their MOTHER—will always be there for them. I cannot assure them that I will be ultimately responsible always. I cannot tell them—because I do not believe it—that they will be all right without me, that my death will not damage them. From my breast, from which has come the milk that has sustained, comes a poison to kill, not just me, but them too. A part of me believes this.

. . . I am sitting in a small windowless room. A person tells me I have cancer. Another person has seen the flesh of my ducts under a microscope and found cancer there. Tiny cells, clumped together, misshapen, diseased. I have no compassion for these monsters in my midst. I hate them.

Days later, Hilary invents screamotherapy. It comes before my next operation, the radiation treatment and chemotherapy. For days my children scream at the cancer in my breast, "No! I hate you!" We learn fifty ways, in different languages, to say "No." Miranda can scream for long periods at a time. Ben, my nearly adolescent child, is more tentative, but equally betrayed. By the time I have surgery, several days later, we are spent from scream-otherapy. But it has done what it had to do. It has enabled us to live in an authentic relation with the cancer cells in our midst. It has helped us with our murderous rage until the surgeon can cut our enemies out. . . .

I am terrified of what happens to children whose mother dies when they are young, not ready. I cannot think for the pain of that thought. The night of my diagnosis, I curl up into the tiniest ball I can make, rock myself, and shake my head. I cannot be what I have been, do what I have done. "I feel *this* small," I tell Hilary, holding up two fingers spread two inches apart. "I want to squash myself out. I've done the worst thing I could do. I can't bear to feel this bad."

By morning I have worked my way to realizing that *I* have not been the agent of this appalling reversal in our lives. Cancer has. Cancer is the interloper in our midst, making pain for all of us. I extend great sympathy to myself. A mother, desperate to do right by her kids, who, by cruel and common circumstances, does harm. Perhaps not irremedial harm, but harm nonetheless, and too early, by my reckoning. Certainly for Miranda. Perhaps Ben is more nearly ready. But surely Miranda. The next night she breaks my heart. "Tell me what it's like not to have a mother?"

Not to have a mother. I have been there too. When I was twenty-seven, my mother was diagnosed with an uncommon form of cancer, not breast cancer. I wrote a short story about what it was like to fear you might not have a mother. It is the counterpoint to my daughter's question. What can I tell her?

"You will always have a mother. Wherever you are, I will be with you as a loving presence whenever you want me with you." Should I say that to her, since it has been true for me? Should I tell her that it's hard? That she is right to fear it, but that it is not happening to her? That she will have plenty of time to think about it? That she may be an old lady before she has to think about it, and her grandchildren can help her? Should I tell her that? Or should I say, Your heart is aching. I'm so sorry you have thoughts like that, and so glad you can tell me. You have a mother. And we are lucky, because I have a kind of cancer from which I can be cured, and you won't have to figure that question out now.

I was twenty-seven and I could barely figure it out myself. I did what I always do when my feelings are most intense: I write.

> My mother is dying. Or she may be. No one really
> knows. She has cancer. Or she may have. 'It depends on
> your point of view.'

It is a poignant story, I think now, reading, as a mother, my younger self's daughter's story—reading it like a text that illuminates the questions I have been posing; reading it with my sensibility as a mother as my first and final filter. In this story I am struggling to work something out. A dutiful daughter, after the shock and pain of learning that my mother has cancer, I begin to suffer terrible, inexplicable guilt. Gradually, in the process of living, talking, and writing, the meaning of the guilt takes form. I surface an interior dialogue that happened swiftly upon learning my mother had cancer. I must have said, "Oh, my God, how will I live without her?"—that most scripted of all lines at the revelation of imminent death—and I must have answered, "You will." For the truly dutiful daughter of the truly ultimately responsible mother, this is surely the unspeakable sin, the unknowable knowledge.

I write myself into a conversation with my mother, which I then show her, and then write about again. Here are a few pages of this story:

. . . I thought, How will I live without her? and I answered myself, "Just fine." The answer made me feel like a traitor. She would be so hurt, so devastated, to see her daughter doing just fine without her. How would she bear that, looking down on me? Her loving me always was one thing, my not needing her quite another.

I punished myself for my deep and terrible secret. I started screwing up recipes. "I need you, Mother. I can't cook." The house got messier. "I need you, Mother. I can't clean." My plants drooped. "I need you, Mother. How does one take care of things?" Why, I asked myself, am I having trouble with these stereotypical feminine tasks? No answer. I asked myself other questions. Incessantly. I wept at the answers, foregone conclusions. How can I bear her death? How will I manage without a mother? Always the same refrain: "You won't. You won't. You won't." But the inner voice contradicted, "You will. You will. You will," it said, creating the need to ask the questions and weep anew.

"Whatever made you think I wouldn't want you to live without me?" my mother asked me. It was May, fourteen and a half months after her initial diagnosis. We were alone in my parents' living room. She had just told me she wasn't sure she'd live to see her novel appear next Spring. I thought my head would explode. "You know," I told her, "this is the first time I've heard you say you think you might die from it." Still "it," but no other pretenses.

"The only thing that troubles me about it is that I don't want to be a burden to all of you. I don't mean suicide. We've talked about that, and if it comes to that we'll all make the decision. I mean *being* a burden."

I could hear a voice in my head say, "Danger. Watch out." I could hear another voice say, "Do it. Tell her. Try. She's a different person now and so are you. You have nothing to lose." I listened to the other voice, the louder voice. "I don't think you have any idea of how you are a burden to us. Each of us. I'm sure you don't have the vaguest idea of how you are a burden to me." My look beseeched her, Ask me; do you want to know?

"If you want to, I want to know."

"What's been a burden to me, what I've really been cruel to myself about, is a thought I've had. I'm afraid you won't be able to stand it if you know. I'm afraid it will really hurt you. It's that I, I, I think I'm going to do O.K. without you. I, I think, I'm going to want to go on living my life. I think I'm going to be just fine."

My mother had come over to me and was holding me. Her eyes were dry. "Kathy, Kathy. If I'm not crying it's only because one's own death is impossible to really believe in. It isn't for you. It's harder that way for you. If I've had one wish in all of this, one wish, it was a wish that it could be a gift for others as well as for me. It has been a gift for me. You know that. I live each day to the hilt. So I take a cab. So I buy a fresh pineapple. It makes me feel good. It does no harm. To hear, to hear that it has been a gift to you, too, I can't ask for anything more."

My mother was telling the truth. She did feel fine about my doing all right without her. However, this did not shatter the merits of the idea of ultimate responsibility itself; I turned it around and made it a proof. The ultimate good job of the ultimately responsible mother is to raise her children to do fine without her. So resolutely did I cling to the idea that a mother is ultimately responsible for the fate of her children that I created an airtight case for myself.

From Ultimate to Judicious Responsibility

My thralldom to the idea of ultimate responsibility has produced disabling distortions. Until I had cancer, I lived with these distortions, not noticing the contortions I had to go through to maintain the fiction that I could be ultimately responsible. After I had cancer, my circumstances changed. Having a kind of cancer for which there is no cure—though some of us are cured—created a challenge to my belief that I had to be ultimately responsible. I could not twist myself inside out to maintain my sense of "goodness," since it depended on my thinking myself at least theoretically able to accept ultimate responsibility until my children were grown. Dismantling this belief, though hard, has been liberating for me, my children, my husband, my family, and my friends.

In place of ultimate responsibility I now think about judicious responsibility. I am ready and able to take this on. Judicious responsibility does not exclude other adults or children from taking responsibility too. Nor does it obscure the responsibility that society has—but fatefully neglects—for meeting the needs of mothers, children, and their families.

Giving up ultimate responsibility with regard to my children in favor of judicious responsibility shifts many aspects of my relationship to them. I have wanted to offer them the sense, so palpable in the lyrics of "Summertime," that "nothing could harm them" with me "standing by." I have wanted to give to them what my parents provided so ably for me.

Yet, thinking back, the sense of comfort that my father's assumption of responsibility provided was distinctly different from my mother's. I was fairly young when I realized that my mother's caring had a quality of anxiety in it that my father's did not. My mother was a marvelous listener, until I began to talk about problems. Then her anxiety that she would not be able to "fix" them got in her way. At those times, my father, who was not notable for listening well, could be counted on. Today I would say that her anxiety was due to her taking ultimate responsibility under circumstances in which she didn't have ultimate authority, control, or the illusion of control.

After my mother died, my father's position with me changed. I did feel his anxiety when I told him about problems, just as I had with my mother. Perhaps with her death, he assumed, at moments, ultimate responsibility and took on with that feeling the tangles that it can create.

Two consultations I did this year illuminate these tangles. In the first, two women in their early forties came to see me because they were having difficulty deciding whether or not to become parents together. Barbara, who had been living with Susan for five years, had previously been married and she had two children who were now young adults. Susan had never been married and was childless. Though she loved Barbara's children, she longed for a child she could raise with Barbara.

Barbara was intensely ambivalent about parenting again. "I just don't know if I can do it again. I feel that the responsibility, that total responsibility, is just not something I want to have again," she tried to explain to us.

"What's the big deal, Barb? We'll just take it one day at a time. You just see what has to be done and you work it out," Susan said in a coaxing, coaching tone of voice.

Barbara was not so easily convinced. In fact, Susan's reasoning infuriated her. She turned to me. "Am I missing something? I feel like I'm listening to my husband telling me 'it's no big deal,' which translates into it's no big deal for him, because in the end *I'm* going to wind up with all the work anyway. Susan makes more money than I do, as Joe did, and I know that when push comes to shove, I'm the one who's going to buckle under and dismantle my current life. It's not fair."

Susan was more disturbed than angry when she replied, "You seem to forget that I'm a woman, not a man. I want a baby now like you wanted babies twenty years ago. I want that total responsibility."

"I think, Susan," I interject, "that Barbara is saying something about how destructive that feeling of total, or what I call 'ultimate,' responsibility was for her in her marriage. I'm not so sure Barbara is going to feel reassured imagining your feeling total responsibility, since she knows what happened to her when she felt that way."

The two women were interested in discussing the situation framed this way: How can two people parent without either one of them feeling "ultimately" responsible? We wonder together what options for working it out are available—and closed—to two women, in contrast to a heterosexual pair. This conversation is ongoing.

In another conversation about ultimate responsibility, I was a consultant to a psychology intern who was working with a family composed of an adolescent girl, her mother, father, and a paternal uncle who lived in the home. The father and uncle excoriated the mother for her mismanagement of the daughter, who habitually ran away from home despite the boards nailed to the doors and windows of her room. The mother was at her wits' end, terrified of the dangers to which her daughter was prey, and furious at her daughter, her husband, and her brother-in-law for their contempt of her. She took total responsibility for the child, and the father and uncle blamed her for the girl's actions. The intern reported with horror that in one family session the mother had said to the daughter, "I'd rather see you six feet under. At least I'd know where you are!"

Though an appalling statement, I feel great compassion for what I believe is the reason behind it. By holding herself responsible and being held so by others, this mother had been driven by her concern for her daughter's safety to the ludicrous twist of wishing her daughter dead so that she would be out of harm's way. The problem in the family reflected the problem in the culture at large. As long as the mother believed she was ultimately responsible, as long as no one in her family believed that responsibility should be shared with the daughter, husband, and brother-in-law, she was vulnerable to feeling overwhelmed. When overwhelmed, this mother, like many others, became verbally abusive.

Furthermore, as long as the mother, her family members, and the therapist held the mother ultimately responsible, they were diverted from attending to those problems in the community that the daughter was also reacting to. No one member of the family had the power to affect these problems alone. Among other things, the daughter was reacting to an environment gone awry. She was reacting to the absence of a responsive school system; the omnipresent threat of violence; the easy availability of drugs; the absence of meaningful work for youth; and the prospect of limited opportunities as she grew older. None of these issues could be discussed as long as the problem was framed as the mother's ineffectual parenting, which she needed to accept responsibility for and improve.

I think that one way parents can start a positive change in families is by sharing responsibility with children. I think it can be done in a way that is respectful of children's developmental and temperamental capacities. More important, I think it can be done in a way that does not sacrifice a child's feeling that someone is "standing by." No child, no person, should have to feel alone. "Standing with" can relieve loneliness as thoroughly as "standing over." As a model, "standing with" is more transferable and has less potential for abuse.

I think that judicious responsibility on the part of parents— from making lunch in the morning for a teenager who is tired and late for school, to helping a ten-year-old remember to take her homework, to letting a library fine remind a six-year-old that books must be returned on time, to always watching a two-year-old in a bathtub, to responding to a crying baby—can permit a wide range of feeling and behavior. None of these things must be done always and none forever. None need be confused with ultimate responsibility, especially if you are clear that you are heading toward collaboration with your child, and toward collaboration with other adults who live with you and beside you in the community.

The kind of collaboration with children that I am talking about can be learned by both parent and child. During the Gulf War, for instance, I was very distressed. I invited Ben to go with me to hear a teach-in at M.I.T. The speaker was impressive and disturbing. There were no early visual images, but the verbal picture he drew was alarming. Ben and I were both upset when we left.

It was an icy night. Walking down the slippery exterior stairs, I became, momentarily, confused about who should be taking whose arm. I thought, He is taller than I am, but I am the mother. I know he is scared about the war, but so am I. I think my foot is steadier, but my heart is pounding and I feel panicky, the way I did during treatment. I'm not sure who is supposed to comfort whom. The dichotomy of the query dissolved as the logic of its expression forced the answer: "Both." We can comfort each other.

The solution seems so obvious in hindsight, but for a moment I was confused. Wasn't I the mother? Didn't that mean that I, I alone, was responsible for his feeling safe in this crazy world we had just heard about so graphically? The irony did not escape me that I was feeling ultimately responsible for his safety— a mere three years away from draft age—simultaneously with feeling extremely helpless with regard to a war I deeply opposed.

I understood that I could take his arm in such a way that I clearly communicated, "I am here for you if you want to steady yourself," but that I could hold it so that it was available to me also. I could ask him what he thought of the speaker's perspective and expect him to reciprocate. I could let him know in the interstices of what I said, by tone and by gesture, that I did not have answers and that I did not think I should have. Rather, I could make it clear that I had a sustained and abiding interest in being with him—steady, trustworthy, and responsible—but not ultimately so. And not alone.

I want him to know that there are other adults besides me who take responsibility. Most important, there is his father. To help Ben know that, I have to let his father in totally. I have to release myself from ultimate responsibility so that I can share responsibility with Hilary. I have to do better than I did at the very beginning of my motherhood.

When Ben was born, it took three days for the hospital's pediatrician to come to examine him. For three days I lay in post-Caesarean rapture, refusing medication so I could handle my beautiful son, the child with such marvelously spiky black hair that the nurses had nicknamed him the Brylcreem Kid. I can still see the doctor take off his little diaper, look at all his limbs, and then place the stethoscope on his chest. How well I remember thinking, He is listening very carefully; how confident this is making me feel. He will take such good care of my baby. And then, Does it always take so long to examine their chests? And then, What the hell is wrong with my baby?

"He has a hole in his heart," the doctor said. "I think we'd better do some tests. I'll schedule them as soon as possible. The hole may be either of two kinds; I can't tell. We'll know after the tests. And I think you had better make an appointment with a pediatric cardiologist."

That's what I heard. Not, "What a wonderful baby!" Or, "You have a healthy baby with a small heart defect." Just, there is a problem. I was absolutely devastated. I was recovering from an unplanned Caesarean section in Boston; my husband was working in a nearby hospital; my parents were in New York; and my baby was screaming in my arms.

I reviewed every week of the pregnancy and convinced myself that the sore throat I had had in the seventh week had driven its way down from my throat to his heart and stabbed a tiny hole in the forming chamber. More darkly, I imagined that the lead shield I had worn on a visit to my mother in the eighth month of my pregnancy had been insufficient to protect him from the radium planted in the lining of her heart. I was inconsolable.

When I reached Hilary, he didn't have much to say: "We'll just have to wait and see what it is." I couldn't believe his calm. He isn't bonded to his child, I thought, searching for an answer as to why only I felt I had been punched in the solar plexus— personally attacked and personally terrified.

We went through the tests; Ben was examined by many doctors; and they all had reassuring things to say. It might take a year to figure out what kind of hole it was, but whichever it was, he wouldn't die in the meantime. Nor would he in the long run: there was a surgical procedure to correct either defect, if that was ever indicated as necessary.

But another hole opened up—one between Hilary and me. I couldn't understand why we reacted so differently. We talked about the advantage his medical background provided, my postpartum vulnerability, my grief over my mother's imminent death, my tendency to worry: all were contributory to the disparity between our responses. We didn't list then what I would identify now as critically important. I saw myself as ultimately responsible for Ben's welfare—regardless of whether Hilary eventually took care of him equally or not. For at the moment I heard that Ben was not "safe," I was the only loving caretaker present. If I then slid into the slot of feeling ultimately responsible, I have to notice that the slot was there—not created by the panic of that moment, but available to staunch it. A fantasy. If I could believe I was ultimately responsible, then perhaps I could protect him from my actual helplessness in this case.

Had Hilary been there when the pediatrician came in, I'm sure the drama would have unfolded differently. But even without him there, if I had believed, because my peers did, that both of us were equally responsible for Ben, I'm sure I would have dropped "ultimate" for "judicious" responsibility. If only there hadn't been that available slot.

But, even though the year was 1976—a politically active year for feminism; a year in which Hilary was doing his third year of medical residency half time in order to stay home and care for Ben—I, not Hilary, felt ultimately responsible and was reinforced by others to feel that way. Though Hilary was a doctor, and though doctors told Hilary what was wrong with Ben, they looked toward me as the person who was going to have to take care of it.

The message was clear, destructive, and wrong. The message was based on the premise that a woman is ultimately responsible because she is responsible for the home and men are responsible for "productive" labor. Life never worked that way, and it surely doesn't now. Consciously, my values and my goals contradicted that premise and yet, unwittingly, my thinking, feelings, and actions perpetuated it. I have begun to resist.

Feeling ultimately responsible myself has not interfered with my being able to spot this attitude as a potential problem for other mothers. Years ago I worked briefly with a family whose youngest, school-age son was severely handicapped. The mother felt overwhelmed by his care and required her older children's help when they were at home. Her husband also helped, but he worked two jobs to pay for the boy's costly medical care.

During the course of the first interview, the mother poignantly described her fear that for the rest of her life she would have to meet a school bus at three o'clock. She imagined her older children gone, her husband at work, and herself on a deserted country road, waiting for a small yellow bus to discharge her diapered, six-foot-tall son. She was massively depressed, furious, and held herself, as she was held by her family members, ultimately responsible for his welfare. The achievement of that short piece of therapeutic work was the mother's decision to get respite care. In our conversations the family developed the idea that the responsibility for Tom could be shared with adults in the community.

Susan Suleiman, quoting Erik Erikson, has written that "in order to relinquish her fantasy of ultimate responsibility, a mother needs 'a conception of motherhood shared with trustworthy contemporary surroundings.' " Suleiman points out ways that the contemporary environment is far from trustworthy, making it difficult to give up the fantasy.

I think she is right. I have taken her thoughts to heart. Each time I find myself feeling ultimately responsible, I try to notice in what ways that feeling represents a collusion with a society that does not want to take care of its members. Instead, it wants to foster a belief that individuals—often women and mothers, at that—can and will provide what care is needed. I am also forcing myself to confront the fact that each time I believe I should be able to find remedies—that I should be able to be a good mother by carrying out my ultimate responsibility—I am experiencing the benefits of my class position. That is, I am not confirming that I am ultimately responsible, but, rather, that I have the educational and material resources to take care of my children. In short, the fantasy of ultimate responsibility is a charm that works for only a few. Like magic, it disappears when the conditions that support it are removed.

Cancer has been a good teacher. Living inside my own body the last few years, it has been impossible to sustain the idea that I could be ultimately responsible. If I lived in poverty, if I were a member of an additional minority group, if I were a religious person, I suspect I would have learned this lesson in other ways. It has been my sustained practice with the experience of little control over my body that has helped me to dismantle the construct of ultimate responsibility.

Oddly, perhaps, it was when I realized that I, too, was part of the "untrustworthy" surroundings—that I might die and "abandon" my children—that my perspective on the matter flipped around. I stopped blaming myself for my limitation and, instead, looked around at what was truly untrustworthy. I decided that any idea that made me part of an untrustworthy surrounding was itself an untrustworthy idea.

I think the first step in my passage to constructing a more liberated mothering was to identify the flaws in the idea of ultimate responsibility. Once I began to know which ideas were failing me, I was able to challenge them. Ultimate responsibility was one. Like dominoes, when one idea fell, other ideas fell. Ultimate responsibility depended on a version of the self that no longer worked for me. I tackled that next.

FOUR

What Is a Self?

Conventional feminine goodness means being voiceless as well as selfless.

—Mary Field Belenky et al., *Women's Ways of Knowing*

Because She Is a Mother

She broke the bread into fragments and gave them to the
    children who ate with avidity.
"She hath kept none for herself," grumbled the Sergeant.
"Because she is not hungry," said a soldier.
"Because she is a mother," said the Sergeant.

—Victor Hugo

Honoring Self, Honoring Other

I have gone through my neighbors' yards to the park that abuts their houses and have found the source of the wild blackberries that Miranda and her friend proudly brought home yesterday. Mine is a solitary mission; I am out before either child is awake. I alone see, as yet, that this day has dawned vividly.

I have a small plastic container with me. As I pick the ripe berries, as they land with a dull thud, as if their fall has been broken and their true sound interrupted, I notice that I have not eaten one. "Because she is a mother," I quote sarcastically to myself, trying, it would seem, to undercut the potential impact of this phrase, recollected from my box of morning tea, which has arrived unbidden in my thoughts.

This must be the way that consciousness is shaped. This must be how, unwittingly, but with full participation, subjective experience forms. If I were not thinking about these issues, would this phrase arrest me as I pick, as berries plunk? Or would it slide right in, fitting into a niche that is already there, carved by just such slipped-in, remembered words. This niche is cozy; even seductive. In my fantasy, the niche is labeled with a hand-embroidered sign: "Selfless Mother."

Am I one? Why haven't I eaten even one berry? I am hungry. I love berries. Yet I intend to share these berries with my children when they wake, probably hours from now. It will be long after any trace of my morning's foraging could be found, and I could keep this precious haul for myself. But I don't want to, and I don't think my desire to delay, to defer, to share is selfless.

I have a plan. I want to put these berries in a purple ceramic bowl and watch their color change when I dust them with sugar. I want to see this more than I want to eat a berry.

I am also happy to reciprocate for Miranda's gift of berries and I don't wish to exclude Ben. So "selflessness" does not aptly describe my actions this morning in the matter of berries.

What if I had eaten them all? What if, while content to eat the berries straight from the bush, I had heard the same refrain, "Because she is a mother"? Would I have withdrawn my picking fingers, imagining a slap to finish off the rebuke? Or might I have said to myself, defensively, "Look, berries are not bread." Or "There are more on the bush." Or even have imagined a scene with the children in which I imply that picking the berries, rather than having them provided, is the real treat. I would tell the children, "Guess what I did this morning? I picked blackberries. There are still tons. Want containers?"

With any of these statements, I would be in an imagined dialogue with the implied idea that a good mother denies herself what she wants—or even needs—and that a bad mother does not. A good mother is selfless and a bad mother is selfish. Within this schema, there is no sense of the complexity of any mother's day; of the minute-by-minute balancing she must do, coordinating her own and her child's or children's needs. Rather, there is a split: the selfish/selfless split.

But enough of berries. The selfless/selfish split captures a critical aspect of my inner thinking about mothers. It is my shorthand way of categorizing my life as a mother, and I have terrorized myself with it. Above all, I have feared finding myself on the selfish side of the split. Oddly, I cannot imagine these categories applying to fathers. Fathers may behave in all kinds of ways, but the idea that influences me seems to exempt them from the selfish/selfless tags. If their behavior were plotted on a continuum, I might label the ends "out of it" and "heroic." I don't expect fathers to be selfless, and when they are selfish, I don't register their behavior as such, because I never had a clearly articulated expectation that they shouldn't be in the first place. Categorizing mothers', but not fathers', actions as either selfish or selfless simplistically caricatures mothers' lives while simultaneously creating a double standard for fathers. Though this way of thinking is appalling, I was under the thrall of such ideas for a very long time.

Thinking according to this dichotomy about mothering has been as confusing and personally wrenching to me as any aspect of mothering. It is the aspect of mothering that has silenced my voice more often than any other. When I might have wanted to say "No" or "Not now," I have said, "All right." In these moments I know that I have met my children's needs as much to avoid feeling bad as to make them feel good.

But why? Part of the quest I have been on has been to understand as fully as possible why saying "no," why asserting my needs, has felt risky. What was at risk? Or, conversely, what was I willing to risk by saying "yes"? Answering this question has led me to understand that historically, at least in the West, the meaning of self-realization has been conceptualized quite differently for men and for women, particularly mothers. I have learned that I have been caught in dilemmas arising from different views of self-realization.

As many writers have pointed out, the Western idea of the self has gone through many changes in the last twenty-five hundred years. There is nothing permanent about our ideas of the self; that is, these ideas change along with other fashions of the times.

According to this view, the way we think of the self is connected to our concept of the individual. Many people believe that the anthropologist Clifford Geertz has best described the Western concept of the individual of the last two hundred years when he labels it "a bounded, unique, more or less integrated motivational and cognitive universe." In other words, the Western idea of the self is that it exists as a solitary, autonomous, self-sufficient entity.

This idea of the individual developed most rapidly during and following the period of the eighteenth-century revolutions. The effect of the revolutions was to do away with hierarchical distinctions, for some people. Hierarchical distinctions were not erased for women, children, slaves, and men of insufficient means; these groups were not accorded the rights of individuals. Individualism, and the notion of the autonomous, masterful self that accompanied it, was not extended to women. On the contrary, another role was carved out for them, that of the mother, and with it another version of the self.

The new concept of motherhood supported the new centrality of the individual, although not by endowing *mothers* with individualism. Rather, the purpose of motherhood was to nurture individualism in others. Mothers were to seek not personal gratification but the selfless gratification of caring for others. It was primarily in the home that mothers were to practice this ideal, by caring for their husbands, children, and property. Clearly, the ideal was loaded with contradictions for mothers who had to work outside the home in factories or other people's homes.

A variety of child-rearing ideologies developed to support this construction of the maternal self. Rousseau's ideas in the eighteenth century contributed to the belief that a mother's selfless devotion to her children was vital for the child's social and emotional growth, and necessary to create a productive citizen. In the twentieth century, psychoanalytic and child-development ideologies describe the "correct" maternal self as an "ever-present vessel for the child's needs and desires, which, properly handled, will enable him [sic] to grow into a happy, well-adjusted adult. The Mother's own needs and desires have no place."

The mother who could be this selfless vessel had to be prepared for her role. She was brought up believing that the ideal of feminine goodness was selfless care for others. She was not reared "like a boy." She was not brought up nurturing her own self. I was.

As I think about it, I see that I was brought up in an era that encouraged individualism. I was treated by my family and by other adults as if I would move into adulthood like a man. I was given educational opportunities that would make this more likely.

At the same time, there was something askew. I know I felt a looming contradiction—motherhood—and I also think I was aware of inconsistencies early on, although I could not verbalize them. I think I sensed that this self I was constructing was temporary—possible until I became a mother. Then matters were going to have to shift. Maybe that explains why when Hilary was ready to have children, I was not. I wasn't ready to give up my self. I wasn't ready to make the trade: a child for me. After all, my mother had instructed me to care about my self.

I have an early memory of my mother telling me the following story. I can't say I remember her story verbatim, but I remember the central line verbatim. She told me that when she was a girl there was a billboard and that on this billboard was a picture of a man wearing BVD underwear. The caption was "Next to myself, I like BVD's best." My mother told me that she couldn't believe that someone could think that she liked herself best!

I found this story extremely confusing. On the one hand, I knew my mother was telling me that, when she was a child, she couldn't imagine someone liking herself best, but that she now could. I knew she was telling me that she could understand if I were the sort of girl who was able to say she liked herself best. In fact, I think the point of her story was an instruction to put my self first. Annotating this story in the light of my current reading, I think she was telling me to take on the Western self of individualism. The story's lessons were not so simple, however, because they were embedded in multiple contexts.

First, the person in the underwear was a man. How did I know it was O.K. for *girls* to put themselves first? My mother seemed to be telling me that it was fine, but I was less than certain. Hadn't my mother found happiness in life, and hadn't she been uncertain whether to put herself first? Was this, perhaps, the better strategy for a girl?

Second, I thought my mother might be giving me a hint: "If you think I'm wonderful," which I did, "the secret of how I got this way is that I went through a process in which first I thought nice girls should never admit, much less feel, that they liked themselves best, that they put themselves first, and then I realized that it was fine to do so."

This left me more confused. Because didn't she like me best and put me first? I actually used to ask her this. "You like me best, don't you?" To which she would heave a great sigh, and allude to how complicated "it" all was, and never answer me definitively.

I was unable to articulate one word of my confusion, for I wanted to be good and to do what my mother would approve and admire. I also wanted to be like her. This created a bind. If I did what she said and put myself first, then I would be good, but not like her unless she put herself first, which, because she was my mother, I could hardly bear imagining she would do.

I think I must have cleared up my confusion by thinking it fine to put yourself first until you became a mother. Then, in that far-off distant future of mine, children would come first. But until that time, I was supposed to care for my self. Doing so wasn't selfish; it was "good."

Carol Gilligan writes about this point in female development. In *A Different Voice* she identifies an ethics of care and an ethics of justice, and suggests that it is crucial to listen to the voices of those who speak using the voice, or language, of each. Discussing her own book, Gilligan wrote that there are problems for female development when "in the name of virtue" females think it fine "to give care only to others and to consider it 'selfish' to care for themselves."

According to this formulation, I managed a stance about caring without serious difficulties until motherhood. Then, the script of motherhood collided with the script of individualism. My mother's BVD story had served me well, if not without some puzzlement, until I became a mother. Then, I was sure I should become like her, a paragon of selfless care.

My first encounter with the dilemma of honoring self or honoring another who is infused with one's self came when I was leaving my first childbirth class, pregnant with my first child. I remember walking away, up Beacon Street, sobbing, feeling trapped by the child within to whom I was already deeply connected, and knowing that the passage out for this child, through my body, would require me to endure a pain I was terrified of and feared I would not be able to bear. Two words played over and over in my mind, like a record with a warp: inexorable and inextricable. I could not figure out how I was going to preserve my own needs without subsuming my interests to my child's. I feared that in temporarily suspending my needs I would lose sight of them. I feared that I would become, not just for twenty-four hours, but for a lifetime, an abandoned self, a person joined with and at the disposal of another, whose interests would so converge with my own—for I did also want what was best for my child—that, like a Moebius strip, I would be unable to tell whose surface was whose, whose self lay where.

Out of the selfish/selfless split that I perceived all around me as a central way of defining and categorizing mothers' behaviors, I created a continuum. The continuum was not an abstraction, but a visual image that would occur to me, sometimes several times a day. I would place myself on it, giving myself high or low marks, depending on where I fell. The line was bounded on one end by selfishness and on the other by selflessness. In the middle, the elusive middle, was a location I characterized as healthy entitlement, self-focus.

I have had an uneasy passage along it. In those years when I believed I was sliding between selflessness and selfhood, I may have felt as if I were going down the drain, but I was certain I was being a "good mother." Following my cancer treatment, when my range covered the entire continuum, I couldn't tolerate my lapses into selfishness. I felt "bad."

Here are two memories, both true:

It is very hot. I am waiting for a bus with my son, Ben, who is two and a half years old. I am seven months pregnant and already huge. My feet are thick and swollen in their sandals, and Ben is hopping in blue sneakers. I am looking down at him. He is hot. He is complaining of the heat. Every pore of me is sweating and wanting to make *him* feel comfortable. I am amazed that this can be so. I think to myself that, in this moment, I am really my own mother in my body. I begin to weep sweet, spare tears. One or two. I feel so grateful that my mother gave to me in such a way that I can now do this for my son. I am so happy that I want to pour every effort into his distraction, for the sake of his comfort, his amusement. I thank my mother silently and tell her that, in this moment, she is helping her great-grandchild, for Ben will store this goodness and, someday, on some block, on some hot day he will bend down and see his small child and pour himself into this child's, my grandchild's, well-being.

I love this memory. I loved the moment at the time. It is very important to me that I was able to mother this way at times. But there is another memory, equally typical.

I am in my kitchen. It is summertime. Ben is ten years old, Miranda is seven. They are each playing with a friend in the next room and I cannot hear myself think. I am frantic. Panic is welling up in me. I want to scream. I want to scream "Stop!" I want to tell all the children to leave, or at least insist that the two friends return to their homes, to their mothers, who are thinking in their kitchens. I am paralyzed. I cannot say a word. I cannot figure out what is fair. I cannot think my way out of this most trivial, essential, and commonplace moment. I cannot decide if I have a right to quiet or they have a right to play, loudly. I think, Your mother would never have told you to be quiet, and I think also, Your father would have. I feel myself utterly confused. My parents' actions are no help to me now, for I know that their circumstances are not mine. I cannot think or feel my way to what I want to do, much less to what I think I ought to do.

Both of these memories can be easily shared, for they conform to ideas that I have held about how a good mother should be. In the first I am unambivalently devoted and in the second I feel tortured by the idea of putting my needs first. The mother's voice in each is acceptable to me. It is another voice, my selfish voice, that threatens me and that threatens others. No one wants to hear the voice that tells her children "No" when they ask her if she *wants* to do something for them. "No. I don't want to." Mothers who express their feelings regardless of their children's feelings about something are infrequently admired. No one wants to know about the times I have heard my child crying plaintively in another room and thought, "Dammit." For many mothers, not just for me, this ordinary, garden-variety voice is unacceptable. As long as it remains so, as long as we hide this voice from one another, we will have no opportunity to understand these experiences of a mother's self.

Self Experience

Perhaps the "selfish" voice remains silent, for those for whom it does, because it cannot exist under anyone else's cover. The selfish voice clearly expresses the mother's subjective experience; it is not a composite expression—part mother, part child—as the selfless voice can be. According to the good/bad categories that have enslaved me, the aims of the good mother are supposed to be close to the desires of the child. Thus, when a mother places her perspective on the back burner and attends to what she *thinks* is her child's perspective, she can assure herself that she is a good mother. However, by taking the child's perspective, a mother risks losing her own self experience. It is not uncommon to talk with a mother whose sense of herself as subject seems vitally absent.

The children's classic *The Giving Tree* provides an uncanny illustration of this point. Although the book ostensibly tells the story of a tree who demonstrates that, even as she ages, she has value to others, the tale actually glorifies the selfless love of a mother—symbolized by the tree—for a young boy. The tree happily supplies him with her bounteous resources—shade, fruit, branches—receiving modest appreciation in return until, at the end, she annihilates herself to gratify and comfort the boy grown old.

The story is described as "tender," a description that only makes sense from the perspective of the boy, who is unable to empathize with the tree. But tender is surely not the word that a mother would use to describe an act of self-sacrifice. When mothers sacrifice themselves for their children, which they do, their emotions are passionate ones. The word "tender" obscures the fact that the tree/mother dies; it only accounts for the boy's experience of sustained caring.

Additionally, the word "tender" may apply to the reader who, infused with the perspective of a culture that wipes out maternal subjectivity, reads the story and approves, feeling glad for the boy and gratitude to the loving, giving tree. Yet, how different the story would have to be to account for the mother's experience of her death. Her feelings have been written out of this story, and out of countless others we read, see, and live daily.

I have erased myself, also, on occasion. When Miranda was born, we were uncertain whether she would live or not. I made a decision to keep a journal about her, as if she would read it one day. I remember how often I wrote a sanitized version of my feelings, willing to trade the fullness of my expression for the hope that she would one day read the entries. The choice was an optimistic one, but it expressed a particular view of mothers: Mothers must keep the totality of their experience to themselves, for they have the potential to hurt their children.

I censored the intensity of my pain, my worry, my fear, and my outrage, for I was unable to imagine a Miranda able to bear knowing that her mother had felt that way about her. I had no idea how I would explain that I felt all that *and* a love as fierce, passionate, and joyful as any I had ever felt. I think I could not imagine Miranda, as a child, understanding me. For if I had thought that my child, as a child, might be able to appreciate who I was, that I could have some part in letting her know me as I would learn to know her, that *my* experience of my self could have as much a place in our life together as hers, I would have kept a different journal.

Two clients come to mind. Both are mothers of nine-year-old daughters. Both mothers were incestuously abused by their fathers and neither mother currently has any contact with her parents. The first mother, Rachel, has never avoided talking with her daughter about her abuse. She had left home and worked with other incest survivors, learning that her experiences were common and devastating. Grieved and enraged, she also saw herself as part of a large, if silenced, group. In the community she has constructed for herself, a story of sexual victimization is dominant.

Rachel's daughter knows why her family visits her father's but not her mother's family. Rachel has given her more complete explanations as she grew older and more curious. She began, Rachel told me, with a statement like, "We don't see my parents because they hurt me, and I'm still angry because they never said 'I'm sorry.'" When her daughter later asked what they did to her, Rachel told her that she was sexually abused by her father and her mother had not believed her. Her daughter has asked her mother what her father did to her, and Rachel has told her that he touched her private parts many times after she had told him she didn't want him to do that.

My other client, Rosalie, has never mentioned a word to her daughter about her parents or her experience with them. Occasionally her daughter will ask if she is going to see her grandparents—before a birthday, for instance. Rosalie has overheard her daughter saying to her dolls, "My grandparents don't like me. They don't want to see me. I'm not going to get a present from them this year." This breaks Rosalie's heart, yet she cannot imagine telling the child what her father did to her. Instead, she remains silent in face of the probes and indirect comments her daughter makes. She diverts her daughter's attention elsewhere, if she must, to keep her away from this topic.

Rosalie thus prevents her daughter from knowing a vital part of her. In effect, she is erasing herself as subject. Yet she does this for a variety of psychologically cogent reasons. First, she fears that if her daughter knows of the abuse, she will worry about her own father's potential to abuse her. In therapy, we have been talking about whether this response from the daughter is really likely, or whether, in fact, her having been brought up to challenge her father when she feels wronged weakens the parallel to Rosalie's life.

Second, Rosalie does not feel ready to talk to her daughter about her experience. She does not want to speak for fear she will be unable to manage the vivid images she will recollect. This reason makes her experience central; her experience of herself counts. For Rosalie, at this time, not speaking honors her current needs and enables her to be the mother she wants to be.

Neither woman has had a good choice to make. Rachel has multiple physical symptoms that she attributes directly to her abuse history. Her daughter seems, at times, serious and concerned beyond her years. She acts protectively of her mother and is vigilant herself about inappropriate touch. Rosalie is often exhausted—not only because she works at a demanding job and then has a child and home to tend. She yawns and feels sleepy whenever the topic strays to parents, sex, or childhood history. Her daughter, who "knows" nothing, knows to step gingerly around certain topics, the categories of which she could probably never name.

Both of these mothers feel doubly victimized: first, by their fathers, and now by having to introduce an incest story into their family if they are going to be fully known. Both mothers feel that the choice to tell or not to tell is fraught with problems for them and for their children. They resist making room for, or feel bad that they must include, this aspect of who they are and who they have been.

Rosalie fears that what she has to say will hurt her child, passing the hurt to yet another generation. She will not do this. Rachel worries that what she has said has hurt her daughter. Both women, though each has handled her situation differently, struggle with representing themselves fully, for to do so confronts them with challenging their children to understand that the world may not be a safe place—that, in fact, home may not be. They would give anything to be able to protect their children from this knowledge, now, while they are still young, and yet they cannot. One daughter knows what's up and the other one knows that something is up. These mothers have dreadful choices. Letting their children know them more fully requires that they also know about the terrible violations certain kinds of love can include.

Shifting from the Idea of a Single, Fixed "Self" to a Coherent Account of the Self

Up until my diagnosis, the way I had thought of a self was as a fixed, coherent, stable, internal structure. When I thought about my "subjective" experience I envisioned my "I," my "self" as if "I" were as simple a form as the letter "I" itself. Partially persuaded by the word "self"—so singular, compact, clear, and defined—I assumed that my experience of my self should be likewise. I accepted the idea that my self was one entity, even though this did not account for all of my experience. It was hard to retrieve the experiences that countered this notion of self, because my idea of how a self should be blocked me from attending to experiences that didn't fit. It was as if these exceptions were stored in an unlabeled box. Each time I went to the shelf to pick out an anecdote about the self, I retrieved the same box, the one that was labeled "The self as one stable, coherent entity." I am trying now to identify frameworks of the self that can account for more of my experiences, both personal and professional. I want to label my other boxes.

Recent work in social psychology and philosophy suggests that there is an alternative way of thinking about the self and subjectivity. Rather than the self's being an entity that develops stability over time, the self is now thought of as a capacity to render a coherent *account* of oneself over time. The self is a kind of telling about oneself. This account is necessarily dependent on one's context, and contexts are various. They include the people with whom one relates and the material conditions of one's life.

Applied to my experience—say, listening in the kitchen to boisterous children—I can understand my monumental indecision in the face of a minor, transient, regularly occurring event. I am paralyzed by my idea of the self, an idea that implies that each choice I make confirms the type of self I am. If I let the children make noise, I am a good mother but a bad individualist. If I tell them to be quiet and ask the two guests to go home, I am a bad mother but a good individualist. I have difficulty making the choice, because these are the stakes.

The alternative view of the self gives me much more leeway. In this framework, my choice does not have to reveal *who* I am. Instead, it can show what I decide to do in this situation, which I then describe in particular ways—either to myself, to others, or to both. With this view of the self, the self is no longer an entity but an account, a narrative, or a story.

In this view, the self is the ongoing story we tell about ourselves, to ourselves and to others. And, just as important, the story we tell about ourselves is influenced by the stories others have told, tell, and will tell about themselves and us. In this sense, then, the self is not fixed and enduring, but evolves as a continual process of telling. We have many opportunities to create coherent stories to account for our feelings, thoughts, and actions.

The ramifications of this shift in thinking about the self are important. When I am paralyzed in my kitchen, unable to speak, I am censoring myself with my children. I am acting as if I believe a good mother should always let her children's stories take priority over hers. I am acting as if I believe that the mother's role is to nurture the child's story so that the child can develop his or her essential inner self, but that *she* should withhold her own story. A good mother is a vessel to be filled with her children's stories, for this is how she promotes the development of the child's self.

Once this view of a fixed self is rejected, the suppression of the mother's story becomes not only unnecessary, but also undesirable. In fact, if we think that the self is a capacity to render a coherent account of oneself, then to withhold from the child the stories of a critical person in the child's life handicaps the child. In the absence of accurate maternal stories, children create flawed accounts of their own and others' experience.

By accurate maternal stories, I do not necessarily mean complete ones. It's not that telling all is preferable to telling some or none, but that believing one has a choice is better. For some mothers, to believe they *do* have a choice means believing that a mother can talk about herself in a way that does justice to her experience without violating the capacity and the interest of her child. Children can be asked to listen to their mothers' experience in a way that does not burden them or exceed their capacity to bear what their mothers might say. However, it must happen in a way that is mutual. It is not the sharing that leaves children feeling burdened as children, and later as adults. It is the particular ways that "sharing" happens that can backfire for parent and child. Sometimes not sharing is more burdensome than sharing. When my son was sixteen months old, that was precisely the judgment I made one morning.

Ben and I were playing in the living room before a trip to see his father's parents. Eager to see them, I was, nonetheless, sad that I would never again plan a visit to my mother. I began to cry softly. Ben looked up from his toys with a look I interpreted as concern on his face. Wanting to be clear with him, I said, calmly, "Mommy's sad." He got up, went into the kitchen, reached up to the counter where his bottle was kept and brought it to me, insisting on pushing it into my mouth. He then went back to his toys, content, I think, that he had made me "all better."

My timing was right. The two words were all I needed to say to express the depth of my despair at that moment. I shared myself with Ben in a way that rendered me intelligible without overburdening him. In fact, I suspect he felt competent and good, able to help his mother. That exchange has always been very important to me. I wanted to acknowledge verbally to Ben what he could see anyway, that I was sad. I had no expectation that he should comfort me, so his gesture was particularly precious for being unanticipated. While I deplore challenging children past their specific developmental or stylistic ranges, I don't think it helpful to underestimate children's capacities to listen, to understand, and to respond to their caretakers, mother or other. The self-contained, storyless mother who withholds her feelings may fit one version of a maternal ideal, but this stance creates difficulties of its own. How do we prepare for our own lives—lives that will be filled with intense feelings and thoughts and experiences—if not by observing the ways our loved ones handle theirs?

My mother struggled with sharing her stories with her daughters. Having been told too much about her mother's life, she wanted to avoid using us as confidantes. At the same time, she longed for intimate connection. Fortunately, she did share a lot of herself with us in a way that felt respectful. On the one hand, I have a better sense of my mother's life than many of my contemporaries have of their mothers' lives; on the other hand, I know from reading her journal that she edited herself in speaking to us. I wish I knew more about how my mother managed the intensities of her emotional life. More than anything else about my relationship with my mother, I regret what she didn't say, rather than what she did.

Two experiences come to mind:

When I was ten, my mother's favorite aunt died. She told me so. Later that day, I came into the kitchen and found my mother crying while she was talking on the phone.

"Why are you crying?" I asked her.

"Because Aunt Peggy died," she replied.

At that point I began to scream and sob and shout at her, "Why didn't you tell me? Why didn't you tell me?" I ran out of the house screaming. My poor mother ran after me, down the asphalt road. When I let her catch me, she said, "I thought I told you. I thought you knew. I'm so sorry; that must have been such a shock."

I let her apologize for the wrong thing. As I ran, I began to remember that she had told me. I let her apologize for *not* telling me, when the problem was that she had told me in a way that did not stay in my mind. She had not put her pain and her sorrow in the telling. Able to conform to the conventions of the day, she, in 1950s style, "protected" me from the rawness of her feelings—so much so that I could not hold on to the fact that my great-aunt had died, much less place it in the emotional life of my mother.

Nor did she tell me in a way that made it clear that something would be expected of me. I was ten; I loved my mother. I would gladly have soothed her and comforted her, and I know she would have appreciated that. But the times worked in us both, distancing us through our conformity to standards that we accepted, even if they weren't all we felt or wanted, and even if we couldn't have articulated those standards.

These same standards continued to play a part, though decreasingly, throughout our relationship. My mother continued to "protect" me from the full range of her feelings, choosing to monitor carefully what she shared. She kept private those thoughts that she deemed "negative" or "critical." It was marvelous and poignant to read in the pages of her journal, published posthumously in her book *Intimations of Mortality,* what she really thought of the story about her illness that I had written.

> . . . And she has our conversations down pat. But what is unnerving—and it *is* unnerving—is to be done to as I have done, to be made a character. She said at the start, "Don't think I know anything you don't, because I don't." Why? She writes of me as if I were dead. As a matter of

fact, the story says, "My mother is dying." It goes on to tell how my behavior last year changed her, freed her, inspired her, etc., and ends (if I remember correctly—she is sending me a copy, and should, because like the patient listening to a doctor after the shock of diagnosis, I really don't remember it very well)—on a very upbeat note. But I am also a little angry (I am being buried) and a little scared (evil eye business) as well as set up (all I have to do is be noble, and I will not be a burden but a privilege, ha!) and put out about the good writing (a compliment to her—a mother preening over a child, a colleague being jealous of another) and disturbed at my disguise being broken (if it's published, as it should be, may well be) and amused (how many disguises do I break!).

Unfailingly kind, unfailingly "maternal," my mother held back from sharing with her daughters the complexity of her inner life. Her vitality, directness, and self-awareness are thrilling and inspiring to me now, but I can also feel the waste that neither she nor I pushed for a fuller conversation about her reactions to my story or, more painfully, to many other life events. She told me she was proud and jealous; they were both compliments, not openings to a dialogue. Immersed in particular ideas about selfless mothers, I didn't project on to her the kinds of feelings I knew that I would have had in her place. Ironically, she did have them, but neither she nor I was able to connect to each other on the basis of this similarity. In general, I think that had I known her better, I would have struggled with her more and adored, though not loved, her less. I am also sure that I would have been better prepared to accept my own feelings and thoughts as a mother, better able to tolerate my own maternal stories.

Experiences like these make me want to rid the word "maternal" of its connotation of one-way giving and open it up to associations of a richer, more varied, and more complex mutuality—one in which the mother's subjective experience is as vital and central in her maternalness as is the child who is reaping its benefit. Adults have ways of sharing their stories that are mutually respectful of each other. I think that it is no less possible for mothers and children to negotiate a balance with each other. It requires walking a line between saying too little and saying too much, between withholding and dumping. It is worth trying.

In my office, I consult on just such "lines" frequently. Ruth, the mother of the seven-year-old who had screamed "I hate you" at the birthday party, was unable to speak to her daughter, Marya, about the pain her shouted words had precipitated because she was unable to imagine how she could share the "truth." Instead, she withdrew from Marya. She knew that to shout back "You've made me hate you too" would not have been helpful. She also understood that the hate she felt was a reaction to how Marya had made her feel. If she was going to share her experience, not her reaction, with Marya, she would have to understand it first. She knew that would take some time. She chose silence and withdrawal over lashing back.

In a therapy session with Ruth and her husband, David, I suggested that it would be useful for Ruth to take as long as she needed to identify what issues had been stirred up by Marya's outburst. But I was also concerned about Marya. I suggested that Ruth might want to distinguish for herself and Marya that there was a difference between what Marya said and how it made her mother feel. It was my hope that by making this distinction explicit for Marya, in language she could understand, Ruth would give herself time to work on her own feelings without fearing that Marya would be worried that she had hurt her mother deeply. I imagined Ruth telling Marya that Marya's apology had helped her get over the hurt that her words had caused, but that her words had made Ruth think about other times she had felt hurt by other people, and that she now wanted to think about those other hurts. If Ruth sometimes looked sad, it would not be because of what Marya had said.

Ruth thought it a reasonable idea. She replied, "I know Marya, though. If I say that, she's going to ask me what other hurts?"

"And you may decide you can start to tell her something about those other hurts, if you know what they are and feel comfortable naming them with her."

"They are about my sister. And what it felt like when she would tell me she hated me, and how unprotected I felt by my mother."

"So you may want to think about whether it feels comfortable telling Marya that her saying 'I hate you' made you think about Aunt Joan saying that to you. You may want her to know that at some point you will want to talk with her about why she said she hated you, but that even when that conversation clears things up, Mommy may still have feelings from the past about Aunt Joan that Mommy will be thinking about by herself."

"Yes. I think I can do that. She knows already I've had hard feelings about Joan. Marya once pinched me and I told her never to do that because it reminded me of Joan's pinching me when I was a child and I was very sensitive to that."

I felt that it was possible to address the mother's needs without choosing between hers and her daughter's. I felt that there were issues of vital concern to all the members of this family and that it was possible for each of them to emerge with strong voices.

It was important for Marya to know that her mother had been very upset by Marya's making a statement *in public* that had reminded her mother of painful experiences with her own sister. Marya needed to know that Ruth didn't blame her for these feelings.

On the other hand, Ruth didn't understand what had triggered such a strong response in her daughter. At some point, she thought she would want to find that out. I supported her taking as much time as she needed to feel ready to inquire about the feelings Marya had had.

In attending to her own needs, knowing that David was there to tend to Marya's, Ruth took care of herself in the context of her own powerful anger. She didn't deny her feelings during this time and she didn't lash out at Marya. She also didn't swallow her feelings in order to "protect" Marya from them. She waited until she could tell Marya the story of her own feelings as she understood them.

In the context of couples therapy, the mother's feelings are likely to be related and responsive to her husband's. In their case, David was able to sit back and let Ruth do her work in his presence, believing that he and Marya would ultimately benefit. Though appreciative, Ruth also believed that David's attentive listening was her due.

I took an active position that Ruth could find a means of sharing her experience, her story, with Marya in a way that would be respectful and tolerable to each of them, and I implicitly conveyed the idea that it would benefit both of them. Not just Ruth, but Marya too.

I tried to work with Ruth as I have worked with myself, to have her consider that the self is not an invariant, fixed internal structure, but a capacity to maintain a coherent account of oneself in diverse relationships, settings, and contexts. This account will change as one has different experiences. The idea of a fixed and stable self fits with the maternal idea that I grew up with— namely, that a good mother will inhibit her story and, instead, attend to her child's. My thinking has changed. Now, I think that it is as likely that a mother will handicap her children if she *doesn't* give them opportunities to know her, as long as she provides these opportunities in manageable, masterable chunks. Children can tolerate listening to maternal voices. Mothers must believe not only that a mother's job is to help her children develop an account of themselves with which they can live pleasurably and productively, but also that her children can be part of her developing account of herself. And that both she and they can gain from this sharing.

I don't delude myself that this sharing is always easy to do. I think of Rachel and Rosalie and I appreciate the difficulties of sorting out assessments of what is manageable for whom. I do not think that telling about one's life experience is invariably productive. A mother who spills too much of her story too frequently may inhibit her children's ability to stay unambivalently open to her sharing. Yet I fear that a mother who does not share her account of herself with her children—in some way, however small, given the amount of time she spends with them—may handicap her ability to experience herself coherently, and eventually her children's ability to understand either themselves or her.

One client, having made the decision to protect her young son from the grief of her several miscarriages and stillbirths, found herself getting fixated on trivial matters with him—like whether his shirt was tucked into his pants when he left for daycare every morning. With my encouragement to share with him in some small but accurate way what she was thinking each morning— she was imagining a breakfast table with five more children— she finally condensed her experience into a simple sentence: "Mommy has a lot on her mind that makes me sad at times, but it's not about you, and I'm so glad that you're here." After telling him this one morning, she felt immediately released from her excessive concern about her son's clothes. She had brought herself more fully into the relationship.

In the last few years, I, too, have brought myself more fully into the relationships with my children. The experience of cancer challenged me in all kinds of ways to identify how much they and I needed to know about my situation—my prognosis, my physical status, and my emotional well-being. For instance, at first, I was comfortable with their being at home the days I had chemotherapy. Toward the end, I was not. My privacy was essential. If I could have obliterated my *own* account of those days and nights, I would have gladly. I saw no need to share this aspect of my life with them. But I emerged from the cancer experience with an urgency to leave a trace of myself; this expressed itself in a desire to record my experience and what I learned from it. Fortunately, I was able to share this goal with my children, and they seemed to appreciate that I wanted to write things down. They have been able to tolerate—show indifference, irritation, and pride—that they have a mother who both writes and works. I would say that, on this score, their account of me corresponds with my most evolved account of myself—

an account I have also had to work on developing. They understand that I am a mother and a professional. They "get" that this represents a totality, not a split, but that understanding has taken me many, many years. I turn to the history of that understanding next.

~

FIVE

Men's Work and Women's Families

Mothers Can Be Doctors

In the spring of 1969, during our commencement weeks, Hilary and I were told a brain teaser in the company of friends: A man and his son were driving a car and they had a terrible accident. The man was instantly killed. The son was taken to the local hospital, where the surgeon who was called to operate said, "I can't operate. That's my son!" Who was the surgeon?

That spring, none of us could answer the question. Finally, one of our friends offered the following solution: "The surgeon was the boy's mother, but she's had a sex-change operation and now she is a surgeon." We all laughed hysterically—some of us with hilarity and others with humiliation. Hilary and I were flabbergasted to recognize the entrenched nature of our sex-role stereotypes. I think it upset us both equally. Several years later, we heard another friend tell us a version of this same puzzle. Only, this time it was a true story.

In graduate school, my adviser was a physician and psychologist who had five children. Her husband was a physician as well. The children had spent considerable time with each parent, both at home and at the office. One day Mary told Hilary and me an anecdote about her five-year-old daughter. "Yesterday, a friend asked Amy what she wanted to be when she grew up. She said,

'A mommy and a nurse.' 'Why not a doctor like your mother?' my friend asked. 'Mommies can't be doctors,' Amy insisted. 'Well, what does your mommy do?' my friend persisted. 'She's a doctor,' my daughter sweetly replied, without a moment's pause to ponder the gap she had just opened up." Amy was operating with airtight compartments.

A decade later, in the mid-1980s, when our children were young enough so that car games on long trips were de rigueur, Hilary and I told them the story about the man and his son, wondering whether it would stump our children's generation. The context was set by the fact that we were playing games of logic. When Hilary posed the "problem," both kids initially looked blank. Then Ben smirked and said, "I thought you said it was a puzzler?" and Miranda chimed in with "I know. I know." The puzzle fizzled. For unlike us, they had grown up in a culture in which well over half of mothers of children, from newborns to eighteen-year-olds, are employed outside the home and one-third of all graduating medical students are female. For them, not only their own mother can be a doctor, like Amy's, but *mothers* can be doctors. What is "out there" has translated into what is "in there"; what is happening in the world is influencing thinking. What was unthinkable is now thinkable.

The Family and Work as Either/Or

In part, what was unthinkable about a working mother was that she would choose to be "bad." Mothers, it must be remembered, by the late nineteenth century, were charged with the responsibility of the home. The ideology of the day pictured mothers—white middle- and upper-class mothers—as happily teaching their children the virtues they would need to be productive citizens. Boys and girls were taught the values of hard work and morality, with the understanding that boys would apply their lessons in paid employment and girls would apply theirs in the home, raising the next generation of children for the same roles. The "good" mother was at home; the "bad" mother away from home.

This either/or split contained contradictions from the start. The good mother who was "selflessly" caring for her children was not "not working." Even in those homes in which the mother had servants, she often had a complex household to run.

And the bad mother, who left her children, invariably did so to earn money to support them. Her work was for family. If a mother regretted leaving her children—often without adequate care—the false dichotomy of work versus family could only add to her feelings of distress. She wasn't choosing work over family; in order to preserve family she had to work. There is no dichotomy at all.

Psychoanalytic and psychological theories, reflecting cultural patterns of the time, produced clinical and empirical research that "documented" harm resulting from mothers who diverted attention from their families by working outside the home. These theories reinforced, rather than illuminated, the erroneous construction of the either/or, family or work, split.

Psychological theories "proved" that mothers are responsible for the psychological well-being and development of children by accepting as valid the belief that mothers are solely responsible for children. A cultural premise slipped unchallenged into a research program and guided its agenda. Not surprisingly, research prior to the 1970s on the effects of maternal employment consistently showed negative effects. It lent "scientific" credibility to sentiments no more rigorous than Frances Power Cobb's statement in *The Duties of Women,* published in 1881:

> So *immense* are the claims on a mother, physical claims
> on her bodily and brain vigor, and moral claims on her
> heart and thoughts, that she cannot, I believe, meet them
> all and find any large margin beyond for other cares and
> work. She serves the community in the very best and
> highest way it is possible to do, by giving birth to
> healthy children, whose physical strength has not been
> defrauded, and to whose moral and mental nature she
> can give the whole of her thoughts.

Mothers had to choose: family or work. Or, more accurately, good mothers did not work outside the home. I grew up with a mother for whom this conclusion produced a series of cascading binds. She knew from her experience with her own working mother and grandmother that maternal employment was not necessarily harmful. She also understood that without their incomes her family's economic situation would have been intolerable—probably more harmful than any unhappiness she suffered from missing her mother's attention. Later, she knew from her own children that under certain conditions, like the presence of good substitute care, there appeared to be no harm done at all. But she knew, too, that the stereotypes and obstacles she faced as a "working mother" in 1951 were problematic.

Faced with her own complex life experience my mother was truly bound. In two pieces she wrote in 1951 and 1953 for a *New York Times Magazine* column entitled "Parent and Child," the contradictions she was dealing with can be inferred. I read these two columns now, forty years later, as evidence of a premise I live with in my own life: prevailing ideology influences our ability to let ourselves know what we know. In my mother's case, I would say that ideas about what a good mother should do, coupled with ideas about work and family that made them separate from each other, eroded her capacity to trust the evidence of her own life—namely, that good mothers go off to work and take good care of their families. I sympathize with her struggle, for it is mine as well.

In my mother's first piece, "A Working Mother's Job and a Half," under her maiden name, she anticipates by nearly forty years Arlie Hochschild's 1989 description of a "second shift." The column reflects the particular prejudice of her day and her milieu. She opens with a telling anecdote:

> A working mother recently asked her 9-year-old daughter Sally how she had spent a day home from school, nursing a mild cold. She was assured that Sally had had a wonderful time. "I listened to those programs they put on for the working mothers," Sally said.

"Programs for working mothers?" her mother repeated in some bewilderment.

"Yes," Sally said, "those plays they put on all day for the mothers who stay home and work."

Sally clearly belongs to the school that considers the lot of mothers who work outside the home sheer escape. She is like the full-time housewife who runs into another mother coming home from her office and says fervently, "You don't know how lucky you are."

My mother is identifying a variant of the seemingly timeless work/family, good mother/bad mother split. When this piece was written, the pejorative language of selfishness, applied to the mother who works outside the home, supported the post-World War II effort to create jobs for returning GIs. The working mom was seen as selfishly collecting the rewards of paid employment for herself, rather than relinquishing them to the more deserving men. My mother is trying to set the record straight, describing the hardships that working mothers face. By depicting employed mothers as working "a job and a half" she was trying to gain sympathy for women like herself who had been employed before the birth of their children and had never imagined changing this aspect of their lives. In her attempt to challenge the perception that employed mothers are selfish, she catalogues the sacrifices that employed mothers make: She smiles and draws a child close when she would really rather say she's tired; short-changes her job by her own standards to ensure her children's welfare; avoids too much responsibility at work and late meetings that might advance her career; lives on two levels nearly all the time, her mind often on home while at work. Ultimately she builds the case that employed mothers are good, because they feel guilty: "Guilt, that still, small nag, makes this working mother wary." To base a case of goodness on guilt is truly a remarkable feat, exposing the distortions that can enter a mother's thinking as she attempts to make sense of the nonsensical either/or, family/ work, good mother/bad mother split.

A Generational History of Mothers and Work

In 1951, when my mother wrote her first column, I, her younger daughter, was four. Perhaps persuaded by the logic of her own words, that was the year she left her full-time job as a newspaper reporter and settled down to being a full-time house-wife—Sally's version of a "working mother." Thirty-two years later, when my youngest child was four, I became interested in tracing the work histories of my mother's female relatives. I wanted to see if I could understand the terrible pressure I felt to stay at home full-time by reviewing their lives.

The women I thought about were my great-grandmother Julia, who died in her late sixties when my mother was in her late teens; my grandmother Elvira, who died at eighty-four when my mother was fifty-nine and I was twenty-seven; and my mother, Violet, who died at sixty-one when I was twenty-nine. As I thought about their lives, I realized I was selecting stories that contained messages about two themes related to the family/work either/or divide. These messages had not always been as vivid and clear to me as the tales in which they were embedded. Rather, the messages had gradually opened, like Japanese paper flowers—all the parts present and ready, waiting for the water of my accumulated life experience to unfurl them.

The first of two main themes I became aware of concerned the relationship between the work women do and the degree to which their husbands support and facilitate it. The second was about whether a woman's work is visible to others. With regard to the first theme, I received a message that women should not merely have equal opportunity to pursue meaningful work, but should also exercise excellent judgment in choosing their hus-bands, screening out men who might interfere with their choice of involvement with work. Important to the second theme was the realization that I had always been sensitized to notice whether my mother was writing. If she was "busy" (never "work-ing"), I knew I could get her to stop by looking forlorn. In many families the distinction between knowing your mother works and seeing her do so is moot or carries little significance. In my family the distinction has been crucial. Starting with my great-grandmother, who worked long hours at a shop away from home and whose work was not observed by her children, the theme has been passed down, alternating invisible-visible-invisible work by generation.

According to my mother, Julia's first husband, my great-grandfather, had been a storekeeper in Budapest. They had had three daughters and lived a prosperous bourgeois life. Julia had married this man, I was told, because he was a good man and would be a good provider. Earlier in her life she had been wildly in love, but she chose to forgo this relationship for a more secure future. When her daughters were still young, and she herself was only in her twenties, her husband died. Refusing to succumb to this tragedy, she chose instead to petition the emperor to allow her to own and manage her husband's tobacco store. Such petitions were rarely granted; hers was. According to all the stories I've heard, she ran the store shrewdly and loved her work.

The next part of Julia's story I "heard" as if it were told in italics, though I am not sure my mother intended to give it special significance for me. It is the part of her story that has worked its way into my consciousness like a puzzle piece, waiting to fit. Julia was a vital person with a talent for managing— her store, her family, her household. Though she was eager to marry again, she was not eager to give up her independence or her business. Her choice of husband represented careful calculation on her part. She chose a dandy, a man over whom most women, upon discovering that their handsome, sweet-talking lover refused to lift a finger to provide for their support, would have collapsed in despair. For Julia, however, he was perfect. He provided her with exactly what she needed—a reason to continue with her work. As my mother told me, Julia cleverly installed a table in the shop so that her husband could "oversee" her activities and talk with her customers. A witty conversationalist, he transformed the store into a salon. For Julia, it was a turn-of-the-century solution to the family/career clinch. For me, the lesson was obvious: Choose wisely.

Julia's story did not end there. She had three children with her second husband and, within a year of the youngest's birth, she was widowed again. This time, she joined the ranks of the large Eastern European Jewish emigration of the early 1900s. In America she found work cutting hair. At first, she managed to take care of her younger children by working in her apartment. In time, she leased a beauty parlor and the children returned from school to the shop. Whereas Elvira, my grandmother, had been taken care of by a woman she called a governess while her mother worked outside the home, her half-siblings were raised by Julia's "third hand" while they played around the beauty parlor.

In her eighties my grandmother described for me in rich detail the apartment in which she had lived in Budapest. By contrast, she could barely remember having been taken to her mother's shop there and knew only in broad terms what her mother's work had been. As a child, it had been invisible to her. In America, she had known her mother's work intimately: why, what, and how. Both images influenced the choices she made regarding family and work.

I know more about my grandmother and her two full sisters than I do about their three half-siblings. Upon arriving in America at fifteen, fourteen, and twelve years of age, the three oldest children immediately went to work in tie factories. Neither as brilliant as her older sister nor as beautiful as her younger sister, my grandmother put together a reasonable life for herself. She worked, helped her mother with the household, bought a hermit or spice cake each day, and paid for an occasional piano lesson. Though she was never a good musician, music made her feel good. She played the piano all her life, never expecting more of herself than enjoyment.

In some ways Elvira was a classic middle child. She adored her mother, who, she believed, preferred her two sisters. Her older sister was an intellectual who studied French over her sewing machine and eventually became a professor of French at a prestigious college. Her younger sister parlayed her good looks, style, and "airs" into a respectable modeling career. Both women married more than once, chose to remain childless, and pursued work of their own during their entire lives.

Although my mother stayed close to both aunts and told me stories about them, somehow I sensed that penetrating their lives would not provide me the clues I needed to illuminate mine. I was never as intensely curious about them as I was about my grandmother. In retrospect, I think that it would have been threatening to learn more about their lives, because they were not mothers, and yet their lives were full and interesting ones. As a young child I modeled myself on my mother instead, and learned that combining family and work meant combining *children* and work. I couldn't afford to let myself know that there were other ways of having children in your life, if that was something you wanted, than having them live in your home.

I don't think I could quite accept that the grandmother I adored thought she lived in her sisters' shadows. However, she believed she married better than her sisters, though in the beginning everyone but the happy couple believed she had married considerably worse.

It was at her piano lesson that my grandmother met my grandfather. At first she fell in love with his voice, for he took singing lessons with a Hungarian voice teacher who lived across the hall from my grandmother's piano teacher. For weeks she imagined the man to whom the voice might belong. Her teacher, perhaps sensing the cause of her pupil's preoccupation, arranged a meeting between the two. Both were in their early twenties and neither had ever been romantically involved before. They fell in love instantly.

As my mother told it, love was about all they had in common. My grandfather William had been brought up in a rural village in Hungary, one of fourteen children in an Orthodox Jewish family. Because of his beautiful voice, he had apprenticed to a cantor, but some of the ritual practices—such as severing the artery on a chicken's neck—had profoundly disturbed him. Finding himself without other prospects, he ran away to his older brother in America. When Elvira met William, he was playing the role of a hurdy-gurdy man in the Oscar Hammerstein musical *The Firefly*.

From Julia's point of view, William was totally unsuitable for Elvira. The Hungarian community disapproved of the match and told William to leave Elvira alone. But the lovers were not to be deterred. They were married a few months after they met, with Julia's reluctant consent given when William promised to leave the stage.

William was a clever man and understood that his wife's attachment to her mother would prove difficult for the marriage. Soon after the wedding, he informed his bride and mother-in-law that he planned to lease a delicatessen in San Francisco that would serve visitors to the Panama-Pacific Exposition. My grandfather won that round in what turned out to be a long series of skirmishes between him and Julia. Elvira, this time and ever after, found herself in the middle. My mother, Violet, was born in San Francisco during the ill-fated delicatessen venture. My grandfather might have learned from his Hungarian chicken days that he couldn't hack anything that involved food. But he didn't, and soon he and Elvira were quarreling constantly. When my mother was barely three, in 1918, Elvira, leaving only a note for her husband, crossed the country with her daughter and returned to Julia.

Within the year, William followed her. He leased a furniture store in Brooklyn and courted my grandmother to return to him with the promise that this time she could keep the financial records. My mother grew up in an apartment over the furniture store her parents eventually came to own. If she wanted to be near her mother, she could slip down into the store and read quietly on a chair in the corner. My mother became her mother's confidante. Elvira would complain to her daughter about having to work all day in the store, about taking care of the house and taking care of the children (a son and daughter were born eight and nine years after my mother). But Elvira worked in the store long after it was no longer financially necessary. Working hard was part of her ethic, and she found a husband with whom it was possible, even desirable, for her to do so.

Although living above the store was not ideal for my grandmother, in some ways I think she liked having her work so close to home. If she had ever resented her mother's long days away from her family (and she never hinted of her resentment to me), her arrangement certainly was a correction. Her children could see her, doing whatever she did, whenever they chose.

Growing up above the store, frequently caught between angry parents, my mother made promises to herself as a child. She vowed she would never fight with her husband, and she didn't; she vowed her work would never intrude on her family's life, and it didn't.

Caught between a doting mother and a distant father, my mother developed a surface caution and inner strength. She was extraordinarily gifted with language, and liked to tell about wandering into the Brooklyn Public Library one Saturday when she was sixteen to find that a scholarship exam was being given. She took the English part and skipped the math. She learned a few months later that she had received a full scholarship to Cornell University.

At Cornell, she had hoped to pursue a career on the stage, but the Depression made that dream impossible. Instead, she settled for another dramatic job, working on a large urban newspaper, where, I understand from my father, who also worked for this paper, she was "a damn good reporter." (My mother was always "a damn good" everything. I think people felt obliged to add the "damn" to insure that no one ever mistook her gentle, thoughtful manner for an absence of passion or courage.)

My parents met at a time in their lives when they were both building promising careers. Supported by the radical left-wing politics of the 1930s (as my husband and I were supported by the radical feminist politics of the 1960s), my parents assumed that my mother would always work full-time. My mother chose a man who, far from being threatened by her intellectual competence, reveled in it. The more, the better. Elvira, rather than treating her daughter's fiancé differently from the way her mother had treated hers, repeated Julia's behavior almost exactly. Initially, my father was not "anything" enough for my grandmother. By the time she changed her mind about him, my father couldn't be won back. At some point in her marriage, my mother made another vow: never to harp on her daughters' marital choices as Julia and Elvira had done. And she never did.

Curiously, the men Julia, Elvira, and Violet married were thought to be poor choices by others who later understood the wisdom of these choices. All three men belonged to a cultural group different from their wives'. Whether this difference was pertinent to the men's comfort with their wives' work, I do not know. Nor did I dare find out. When I chose my husband, I continued this pattern.

During World War II my mother worked full-time and was a devoted parent to my older sister, who was born ten weeks before my father left for a three-year stint in the Navy. After my father returned, my mother continued to make most of the logistical arrangements, which, from her description, were awe-inspiring. My mother was afraid that my sister and I would suffer from her employment, so she arranged that when she was home she would have nothing else to do but be with us. This meant that her forty or so dollars were largely paid out to the three people she hired to make her attention to us seamless: she hired a baby-sitter, a housecleaner, and a cook who came at 5:00 PM and left at 7:00 PM to work in our four-room apartment. My mother did errands on her lunch break; took her sick days to care for us if we were ill; and somehow got to our school events and doctors' appointments. I remember those years well, and I remember them fondly. I used to wait for her to come home from work, but I have no memories of seeing my mother work, or even of going to her office. Like Julia in Budapest, but unlike her own mother, my mother kept her work strictly segregated from her family.

After my mother's first column about parenting appeared in the *New York Times Magazine,* she quit her job. "The challenge for me," she had told me when I was old enough to ask for a thorough explanation, "was to see if I could handle being at home full-time without doing work of my own. Nothing else was a challenge!"

The switch was difficult for me. I never told my mother, but I felt that it was my responsibility to justify her being home. I

felt that I had to provide her with something to do. I understood
that she had quit work to be with her children, and I took that
quite literally. I had trouble believing her when she said it was
fine for me to visit friends' homes.

Two years later, in 1953, she published her second piece in
the *New York Times Magazine*. It was entitled "Case History of
an Ex-Working Mother," and her intention was to "report on the
experience of one working mother who heeded the experts and
decided to stay home." Although she writes as if she wants to
believe that staying home has been better for her and for us, the
majority of her points favor the working mother. The piece is
odd. Since she wants to conclude her column in agreement with
the experts of the day, she must say she is happy, when she is
not, and that we are better off, when we are no different.

Knowing what came next in her life—knowing that shortly
after she wrote this piece she gave up trying to be a mother the
"right" way; that, instead, she worked "mother's hours" (making
her writing invisible to us and becoming instantly available, with
a cover on her typewriter, the moment we walked through the
door); that she never gave up her work again—it is easy for me
to interpret the endorsement she gives to being a full-time
mother as only lukewarm. "Having tried both ways," she wrote,
"certainly at this stage of our lives, it seems to me that bringing
up your children yourself is the better part. Therefore, I think it
well for girls to be as aware of housekeeping as chemistry. This
does not mean that I think that any mother who stays home is
necessarily a better mother than one who works. Staying home
does not wipe out faults, nor going to work erase virtues. But
given the choice, it seems to make more sense. Certainly I feel
that I am now a better mother. I know I am a happier one." And
then she started writing again, at paid wage-earning work.

In my mother's case, I truly believe that if there had not been
experts touting the negative effects of maternal employment on
children she would never have left her job. Further, although
my father was skeptical about her employment causing any
problems for us, her job became inconvenient for him as he became more successful. He had done the morning shift at home,

which meant that he couldn't schedule meetings until 10:00 AM. Even in the 1950s there was some cachet for him in this idiosyncrasy, but not enough to offset the trouble. I suspect he was ambivalent about her decision to quit work outside the home. I suspect that they, along with countless others, colluded in presenting the explanation that she was home for the sake of the children, when in fact she was at home as much for his convenience as for our benefit.

Soon after she stopped her job, she became bored. She began free-lance writing, but, true to her vow, she never allowed it to impinge on us in any way. I knew she wrote—she frequently had projects set up in two typewriters in our house—but I never saw her type. When I opened the door and cried out, "I'm home," my mother became instantly available to me. I never knew how deeply she cared about her writing and didn't understand that her "vagueness" was preoccupation until I left home.

When I went to college, I thought my mother was going to be lost without me, bereft because her last child was away from home. I was totally surprised when I learned that, within months of my leaving, she had completed the manuscript of a novel! My mother was fifty that year, hardly the age when men, or women, announce to themselves and the world that they are now serious writers of fiction. But she did.

In my family it was assumed that I would have a career. I always hoped to have a career and I always hoped to have children. I wanted to have a profession that wouldn't require that I compromise my standards for the one with my standards for the other. During college, I stopped premed studies because the problem of expressing my double ambition seemed insurmountable. I, who was used to women doing their work in and around houses and family, couldn't imagine how to nestle a medical practice into a corner of my house.

Initially, I also chose the wrong man. I vividly remember a telephone conversation with my mother during which I complained about my boyfriend. I said, "He has no patience for the amount of time I'm spending on political work. He thinks it's taking too much time away from him." She said, simply, words that even at that time I heard as wish, command, and permission: "Why can't you be with a man who'll think your work is as important as his?" Within a few months I had started to date Hilary. We married two years later.

"Why can't you be with a man . . ."

As it relates to the work/family theme, my history with Hilary divides roughly into periods, two marked BC (before children or before cancer) and two marked AC (after children or after cancer). Before children, we led roughly similar lives. We both worked full-time. I resisted the pressures to be a medical wife and I held Hilary accountable as my partner. Even if he was exhausted during dinner, I encouraged him to talk with me; I insisted that he do a share of the housework; and I made sure that we stayed emotionally current with each other. I didn't have to fight hard for all of this.

The principle was anomalous among our medical friends; I thought I was very understanding of Hilary, but in a different way. I did not take care of him, but then, we both remained able to care about each other. Others, I'm sure, thought that I was a "bitch." On the other hand, the day internship was over, Hilary and I were still married, still fighting, still talking, still making love, and we had no catching up to do with each other.

We had decided to postpone having children until after the most difficult years of training were over, so that Hilary could share more equally. We were both convinced that this was important for many reasons. My parents had shared baby care during my first few years—not equally, but more than most parents in those days—and I believed that this experience had been strongly positive for me. The zeitgeist of the times, the mid-1970s, favored equal parenting. Having done my dissertation on two-career couples, I was clear that I didn't want to become one of the women in my study who had given up the work they loved to tend children they loved. Only the logistics of having a child was an issue with us. And then my mother's cancer.

My mother learned she had cancer (although she may have suspected it earlier) with my father, my sister, and me at her bedside. Her doctor told her good news and bad. The bad news was that she had cancer; the good news was that she would not die right away. She didn't miss a beat. "You mean I'll live to see Kathy's children?"

I was devastated. It was 1974, and Hilary and I had hoped to wait another year before trying to get pregnant. I called and told him what she had said. "We'll do whatever you want," he said. "Whatever you need to do we'll do."

Hours later, I was getting ready for bed in my old room in my parents' house. My father came in and we hugged each other, sitting close together on my bed. "Dad," I said, "you heard what Mom said. Do you think it really matters to her? Do you think Hilary and I should try to have a baby right away?"

My father held me close to him and said words for which I am enduringly grateful: "When it comes to you and Hilary, her cup is full. Do whatever is best for you."

We waited until 1975. Hilary arranged to do his last year of training part-time (three eighteen-hour days), and when the letter of agreement came from the Board of Internal Medicine addressed to *Ms.* Hilary Worthen, I told myself that he was finally reaping the benefit of his name. (The supportive Chief of Medicine at his training hospital told him not to bring the "Ms." to the board's attention.)

There are two stories next: his and hers. Though I know his, and it is tempting to tell it, his story belongs in a companion volume about fathers. I can only tell my own tale. Ben was born in May, and I started back to work full-time in September, teaching psychology at Wellesley College. It was my second year there. Hilary stayed with Ben on Tuesdays and Thursdays, and we had a marvelous woman, Joan Oleson, to care for him five hours a day on Mondays, Wednesdays, and Fridays. Technically, Tuesdays and Thursdays were my "long days" at work.

I soon learned, however, that despite my intentions I was unable to stay away from Ben. I would become distracted at work.

I would tune out my students and imagine myself at home. My milk would let down. I never had the idea that Ben needed me or that Hilary did. Rather, early in the semester I developed the idea that I simply couldn't tolerate being away more than five hours at a time.

I remember walking with Ben in a backpack through the streets of the North End of Boston with my father and telling him that I was leaving academia. I remember his listening respectfully, but asking the kinds of questions one asks if one wants to be sure the other person has considered all the alternatives. Being a grandfather, loving Ben, had not made him deviate from his core position about me: take care of your own needs. This message, delivered consistently throughout my life, was as anomalous in the context of being a new mother as it had been in some situations when I was younger. He had played baseball with me for hours, for example, and he had insisted, when my seventh-grade boyfriend and I broke up, that relationships with men were not the most important things in my life. He was hard to interpret back then, but not now.

On the other hand, I was sure that my mother, who had died shortly after Ben was born, would have understood the conflicting pulls. I believed she would understand that, without my willing it to happen, mothering had transformed me. My wants, my desires were changed. I dreamt Ben's dreams; I felt Ben's pain. I was merged with my son in an empathic fusion that nonetheless allowed me a full range of flexible behavior elsewhere. My relationship with Ben could not be mediated by Hilary's fine fathering. It mattered immensely to me that Ben's time with Hilary was wonderful, and different from his time with me, but it did not make me feel free to leave him more.

My realization of this bind went against the grain of what I thought I had wanted for myself. It was difficult to explain to people who interpreted the feminist proposal for shared parenting as meaning that the mother should regularly leave children with the father, rather than that fathers should also parent. Nevertheless, the latter approach set the pattern of our next ten years.

I see now that my desire to be at home with Ben was not just a longing to be with him, though that is how I explained it to myself. I was also rescuing Hilary from an untenable situation. In 1976, our community was not ready for dads to stay home. Only years later did I realize the important omission in my mother's sentence to me about a husband. Although she had been progressive in suggesting to me that I should be with a man who would value my work as much as his own, she did not say, "Why can't you be with a man who'll feel that being at home with the children is as important to him as it is to you?" because neither she, nor I, nor any of our reference groups could have thought that. Nor, frankly, could Hilary and I have found out whether he was such a man, because his fathering of Ben was so dramatically influenced by the negative responses he encountered everywhere he took Ben during the week—on days when he should have been "working." In contrast to my enjoyable times with other mothers and their children, Hilary was a virtual isolate, at best.

In those early months of Ben's life, Hilary's private time with him was wonderful and his public time was hell. Women, not always the mothers of the children they tended, ignored him. No one ever sat on a bench beside him. Not infrequently, a woman would challenge his caretaking, for instance, whisking Ben off a slide Hilary had let him use, insisting that Ben was not ready and implying that Hilary was incompetent. He hated his year at home. Isolated, knowing no other fathers who were staying home with infants, finding no mothers interested in including him in their socializing, he certainly didn't make me feel that I was leaving a contented duo at home.

I knew all this, but I allowed myself to believe that my sole motivation in risking being "politically incorrect" was that I just didn't want to be away from Ben. I refused to be silenced by the correct feminist position that I myself had articulated along with so many others: Equal parenting is the answer. I articulated my revised feminist position. In a letter to *The Family Therapy Networker,* commenting on the work of the Women's Project in Family Therapy, I wrote:

> . . . They expressed the view that men and women in fam-
> ilies should have an equal opportunity to feel competent
> and to give and get support. Nowhere in the interview
> did these wise therapists suggest that there was one right
> way for men and women to organize their work and fam-
> ily roles. . . . The beauty of this view is that it turns our
> attention away from what men and women do and di-
> rects us to look at who chooses and who supports the
> choices, and in what ways. Men and women need to
> work out with each other how each realizes his or her
> goals and dreams. It is the mutuality of this process that
> should concern us as therapists, not the content of what
> couples select. . . .

I was writing out of my own experience. I felt clear that our
arrangement was one that both Hilary and I wanted, though it
was not the arrangement we had imagined for ourselves. Not
that Hilary didn't share parenting, but I became the primary parent. He and I both cared for the children, but I was the one who
remembered what had to be done. When he came home from
work, he was capable of doing everything there was to be done,
as long as I oriented him. When I came home from work, Joan
Oleson would give me the day's report, and I knew how the
report fit into the overall schema of our life. Hilary did not hold
this particular blueprint in his mind.

For years we fought about whether he had the capacity to
create and update this blueprint. He argued that he did not—
that he didn't have a plan for his work at the hospital either. I
argued that if I weren't around, he would soon develop a
childcare schema. In those years, I did not threaten to give him
an opportunity to find out.

As the children grew older, my internal configuration shifted
too. As Ben turned nine and Miranda entered public school, I
could feel a readiness to move on with my work, to take on
more, to write again. I had coauthored a book that was published in 1982, but I had written from 8:00 to 11:00 PM, after
the children were safely down for the night. I had vowed never

again to write by using my prodigious self-discipline. Instead, I wanted to realign our priorities so that I could work differently.

Unfortunately, Hilary's job did not have the flexibility he needed to accommodate my changing needs, and for the next three years I was the kind of second-shift wife who complains, challenges, and fights for change, but who settles for apologies and promises. I was not silenced the way some of the mothers in *The Second Shift* were silenced. Arlie Hochschild writes that "many women struggle to avoid, obscure, or mystify a frightening conflict over the second shift. They do not struggle like this because they started off wanting to, or because such struggle is inevitable, or because women inevitably lose, but because they are forced to choose between equality and marriage. And they choose marriage." Though I was not silenced, I silenced a level of discontent I did not allow myself to know was accumulating. I, too, would go through the mental calculation about the struggle versus divorce, and I would always choose marriage, because I loved Hilary—though it was clear that I hated the inequalities of marriage. I found it difficult to consider divorcing someone against whom my chief complaint was that neither I nor the children had enough time with him. Instead, I fought him and told him how unfair our situation was, and he agreed and changed a little. The modest changes he made never seemed to fit his awareness of my situation and his fundamental agreement with my endlessly repeated statement "But it's not fair." In our story, we were baffled by this repeating feature for years, until our second AC, after cancer.

When I got cancer, Hilary was there. He was there for me, for the children, for our families, and for our friends. We made a decision that, in order for him to take care of us, he would have to take care of himself; so, in addition to taking on much of my load at home and continuing with his job, he built in a daily exercise program, and he began auditing college courses for pleasure. My year of treatment was a "great" year for him in many ways, not including, of course, the most basic.

Ben told a teacher that he felt guilty that the year was so good for him, considering how horrible it was for me. He didn't realize, and neither did we, that the reason was that, for the children, Hilary had come home. He was home by 5:30 or 6:00 and he remembered their schedules. He drove places, did errands with them, played games, horsed around, and was your basic available parent. Everyone wanted time with Hilary. At some point, I realized that I was distancing myself too much. I moved back in, and the four of us had a wonderful family life, finally, scheduled around the calendar of my debilitating treatments that blasted huge holes in our months.

One year after my diagnosis, Hilary's partners informed him that his lenient time was up. Now that I was better, he had to be fully productive again. Grateful for what he had done, but still unable to function with vitality, and not recovered emotionally, I went into a deep silence. I recovered my voice as a writer first.

In that process, I realized that our second-shift contract had to change, and Hilary realized it too. He announced that he was leaving medicine to become a high-school biology teacher.

In the months that followed, in trying to understand Hilary's declaration about leaving medicine—an idea that he has not acted upon—we have come to understand that hidden in our "second-shift" family are the contexts of the workplaces with which we are associated. They have set limits on the kinds of flexibility each of us has had to offer.

Hilary's heart and mind have been committed to our family and committed to issues of equity, but the practice of medicine in a partnership model is one that requires open-ended, not shift hours. The year I was sick, Hilary's partners granted him an extraordinary favor: they enabled him financially, logistically, and emotionally to feel self-respecting doing shift work. His hospital colleagues also supported his curtailed hours. Everyone appreciated that he was in battle and was needed elsewhere. Once the treatment was over, he turned back into his own version of Cinderella, working his own brand of on-call seventy to eighty hours a week, for a salary that did not exceed what he would make as a high-school biology teacher in our community.

This is what Hilary's declaration of leaving medicine meant: "If I am going to share equally with you, if I am going to be available to support you through the periodic crises of your chronic medical care, I will give up the work that I have loved; I will do shift work, work that has fixed hours, so that you can have the chance to do work with open-ended hours."

This story is not finished, so I cannot tell you the ending. However, when I teased Hilary that I wanted a separation so that for at least three days each week I would not be responsible for childcare and householding (and that he, not I, could have the house), he did some major restructuring of the "management systems" in our life. I made it clear that I didn't want a divorce, just relief. He and the children were going to have to figure out how to do what I had done for so many years. They bought a huge board and four colored markers, a message system, storage bins, and four in/out boxes, which are still in use. They help.

Changing Men's Workplace

My mother's sentence, spoken in 1967, advising me to find a man who would think my work as important as his, condensed a critical theme that had passed down through the generations in her family. This theme expressed a strategy the women in my family had developed to deal with a cultural belief that portrayed women's place as in the home. Finding that they enjoyed working outside the home, even when that work was difficult, they needed to ensure that their husbands would not threaten their ability to do so if, for instance, it should come to pass that their income was not needed. Their solution—find a man who will be supportive of your work—is an adaptation, not a challenge, to the cultural belief. As such, it was pragmatically useful in a limited way.

This adaptation could not, however, solve all the problems that the women in my family, including myself, encountered in trying to combine family work with paid work. The principal problem, of course, was that the women added another full-time job to their existing jobs as mothers and householders, and this was often too strenuous. Their strategy did not address this situation. Nor, interestingly, did it account for the actions of my mothers' aunts, who did not choose lives for themselves that depended on their husbands' good will. They married, but they made their own decisions regarding the work, travel, and leisure they desired. They were liberated women, much loved and valued by my mother, and I still wonder why I never, until now, made their lives part of my legacy. Perhaps it was because there was a hidden injunction in my family's variation on the cultural belief. Embedded in the family's message, and lived out by the women who heeded it, myself included, were two assumptions: that we would have children, and that although we had the right to work, ultimately we were responsible for family.

For many years, my mother's advice seemed to be enormously helpful to my women friends who were contemplating marriage. I would tell them what my mother had said to me, and they, as I, would be grateful and admiring of her wisdom. We believed that she was cluing us in to the secret for which we were all looking: how to combine family and work; how to avoid the struggles we saw all around us. We, ourselves and our husbands, who were radicalized by the feminist movement, sincerely wanted to build egalitarian marriages and families, but we were having a very hard time.

Unfortunately, my mother's advice—like the strategy it represented—was insufficient to accomplish all the hopes we had loaded on it. It did, after all, maintain the false dichotomy of family and work. It also implied that mothers could have it all, if they found men who were content with their having it all as long as they did it all. In other words, the advice liberated a mother for work of her own, without relieving her of the responsibilities of family. My mother's sentence could only take us to the edge of where the culture had come. It would require new thinking about the relationships among work, family, mothers, and fathers to push any of us over into the promised land of full equality. My mother died before she had a chance to explore this edge; I hope to live to name it and do something about it.

As of now, my advice to Miranda about combining family and work will be different, and longer. As of now, though she isn't asking, my sentence will be, "If you are going to be with a man, be with one who will think that your work is as important as his; who will think that family is as important to him as it is to you; and who will work at a job in which his bosses and his peers believe that fathering is as important as mothering and support that belief." I will also ask her to keep in mind that the stresses she and her husband will feel will come as much from living in a society that makes fewer commitments to helping families than any industrial country in the world as from any other causes.

To Ben I will say, "If you marry, I hope you find a woman who will think her work is as important as yours; who will think it as important for you to be involved with your family as it is for her; and that you will choose work in which the values of the workplace, and all those who are there, support men and women equally on the job and with their families." And I will tell him, as well, that he should look to the wider social context of his life to understand the reasons why combining work and family are stressful.

Further, I will tell them both that the families of gay men and lesbian women may have come up with solutions to the very problems with which they and their partners will be struggling. For these families, unable to distribute work on the basis of sex-role stereotypes, may develop strategies that are useful for het-erosexual couples to consider.

Sometimes families do develop alternatives to ideas that are dominant in the culture. For a time, my mother's simple sen-tence was more radical than anything I was picking up from the culture at large. Sometimes it is the wider culture that offers alternatives to the straitjacketing ideas and values found in cer-tain families. I have friends who have found more progressive ideas in magazines, for instance, than in their homes. And some-times it is the people who feel marginalized by the mainstream culture—people of color, people with different abilities, homo-sexual couples—who produce the most flexible alternatives to confining ideas and values. I hope we can be open to all resources, wherever we find them.

Though this chapter has concerned itself with one family's personal history, our history is not an idiosyncratic one. In reading the social science literature on family and work, as I have for the last twenty-five years, I find our experience well represented in it. The current dissatisfaction I feel with regard to the distribution of time Hilary and I spend on family and work is fairly typical, but so is Hilary's belief that his male colleagues don't seem to have such dissatisfied wives at home.

Actually, according to Joseph Pleck—who has done as much social science analysis of the relationships between paid work and family work as any scientist—about one-third of wives are dissatisfied with their husbands' rate of participation in the home. The other two-thirds, he suggests, might want more participation if they believed, as I do, that their husbands had the skills and abilities to be as competent at householding and childcare as they. Pleck offers another reason for the fact that the majority of wives are not dissatisfied with what their husbands do at home, one that I have written about extensively: "Perhaps the most important reason for wives' low rate of desiring more from their husbands is wives' and the larger culture's belief that housework and childcare are ultimately wives' responsibility." It is this cultural belief that will have to give way to other more diverse views before men and women will be able to create equal lives for themselves and their children.

But something other than this cultural tenet must change as well. Pleck cites an interesting and puzzling finding. In large survey research, gender clearly exerts a powerful effect on family work. Women are doing more family work than men. But men's ideas and values about what men and women should do at home and at work, what researchers call their sex-role ideology, contrary to expectation, does not have a consistent effect on men's actual family work.

Though counterintuitive, this fits my experience with Hilary precisely. If our experience is one from which one could generalize, then I have an idea about where to look for the factor that *would* show a strong correlation with men's family work. If I were designing the study, the variable I would study would be men's perception of the attitudes of their workplace, both institutionally and as a group of people, bosses and peers.

I truly believe that if Hilary worked in a profession in which the norms were to limit one's work on the job to allow full and equal participation at home, he would gladly do so. However, he works at a job whose dominant ideology in some key respects mirrors that of the dominant ideology of mothers within which I operate. That is, he is trapped by the idea that, as a family practitioner, he is supposed to give selflessly to his patients and he is ultimately responsible for their fates.

So, oddly and ironically, he and I are both mothers, but he mothers his patients and I mother our family. And just as I can become enraged at him for those times he does not support my efforts, he gets upset that I don't support him in his work. In essence, our conflicts boil down to my wondering why he can't be more available as a father, and his wondering why I won't be more of a wife. These two related roles have their own connotations, and it has become clear to me that I cannot move on with my goals for myself until I am clearer about how I define "wife" and "father."

SIX

Refusing to Be a Wife

My Version of Wife

I was a wife once, for about a week. It happened like this. Hilary and I had rented an apartment in May of 1969, several weeks before we got married, and we worked hard to fix it up, removing wallpaper, painting rooms, sanding floors. We did these tasks in our characteristic ways: I would adequately paint the walls in two rooms in the time it took Hilary to paint perfectly the moldings in one. It was a grand time, making a home together.

By July, we were married, I was working, and Hilary had begun taking premed courses, although he had been a Greek major in college with no intention of going to medical school. Typically, I would come home first and sort through the mail, sit out on the porch, read a book, unwind, and more or less wait for Hilary to return. During the week I was a wife, I changed my routine, as if possessed, which is, of course, exactly what I was. Arriving home, I donned an apron, headed into the kitchen, and began making dinner, starting with hors d'oeuvres—those small slices of delight that, as a child, I used to pass around at my parents' parties. They were my quintessential sign of adulthood and wifeliness, for in my recollection only my mother had ever made them.

Hilary was nonplussed and uncomfortable with my service. Politely, after a few days when "playing house" did not seem to be an adequate explanation for my aberrant behavior, he asked me whether I thought *he* wanted me to wait on him? I answered honestly that I hadn't really thought about him. In fact, I hadn't really *thought* about anything. It was more that I had been overtaken by an idea I had formed in childhood that had remained intact, apparently, after other ideas had formed and transformed regarding what it meant to be a wife, or, more particularly, what it meant to be married to Hilary.

Sometimes I wonder how our lives would have unfolded if, instead of disliking the change, Hilary, too, had harbored an idea of "wife" that meshed with my own. How long might it have taken me to realize that my sweeping and cleaning and cooking and tending and deferring were vestigial reminders of what I had seen but wanted no part of myself? For I had said, quite consciously for many years by that time, that although I wanted to marry I could think of nothing worse than becoming a wife.

Growing up in the fifties among middle-class, predominantly Euro-American families, I saw around me, as well as in my home, a version of wife that terrified me. Wife to me meant deferring, putting one's husband's needs and desires ahead of one's own. Yet I didn't just happen to notice this; my observations were also directed by my parents. Both, but particularly my mother, made me sensitive to issues of silenced voice and limited opportunity. Where my mother and others experienced constraints, my parents helped me notice them. Long before I had ever heard of Ibsen, my mother used to say, in a way that made me know she approved of the women of whom she spoke, "There goes a Nora slamming the door!"

So I couldn't fail to observe that my mother, too, might have a door to slam. But she didn't slam one. Did *she* think she was trapped? There were times I saw her as a bird whose wingspan was too large for her cage. She often hopped when it was clear she knew how to fly. I was aware that she found ways to fly out of the cage, but these flights away were always brief and, to my knowledge, were only in the service of her professional life.

The nature of her cage was always a mystery; I couldn't see the ideas that formed the bars. I couldn't find the source for what dominated her. Looking for clues in my parents' relationship, I found only ambiguous ones. The terms of their arrangement were difficult to decipher. My father and mother behaved as intellectual equals, though he, not she, had the primary career. My mother appeared to wait on my father—she met him at the commuter train; she had his dinner prepared—yet he didn't seem to demand service from her. He clearly had high standards for householding, but he didn't want her to do housework. Their lives revolved around his commitments, not hers, and yet he always pushed her to do more outside the family than she thought she should. She was the one who displayed the outward signs of devotion, and yet I sensed that she held something back.

My parents disparaged wives, but my mother seemed to be one. They talked freely of marital inequity, but I remember no mention of theirs. I could see my mother's submission, but my father's dominance was not knowable. It was as if it were expunged from the record. Yet it is dominance, not submission, that is toxic to me—my own and that of others.

I have steadfastly, consciously avoided domination in my life, but there have been times, which I can see, with hindsight, when I made myself vulnerable to it. If I have succeeded more often than not in avoiding domination in marriage, I must credit the Women's Movement, whose second wave coincided with my young adulthood; Hilary, who wanted a partner only; and my upbringing, in which I was explicitly groomed not to serve a man. When I have failed to avoid domination, I believe that my vulnerability was caused by what I witnessed at home and was constrained from commenting on by both my mother and my father. Silencing sealed my vulnerability.

Domination can be unmistakable and brutal. It can also be tricky and subtle. In this chapter, I will describe the less obvious forms of domination that I believe are pervasive in many relationships, including marriage. Specifically, I will discuss the ways people's thinking can be subtly controlled. By focusing on this aspect of domination, I am not straying far from a root meaning of the word "dominate," namely, to be lord and master. I am focusing on how people establish themselves as lord and masters over meaning, rather than on the ways they establish themselves as lord and master over others' bodies by acts of physical violation. I am certainly aware, of course, of the ways in which these two processes intersect.

Distinguishing Women as Wives from Women as Mothers

Reflecting on my thoughts and feelings about domination, I have found a distinction proposed by Miriam M. Johnson, in *Strong Mothers, Weak Wives,* very helpful. She distinguishes between women as wives and women as mothers and argues that male dominance is more tied to the role of wife than to that of mother. She disagrees with those feminist psychoanalytic theorists—for instance, Dorothy Dinnerstein and Nancy Chodorow—who have identified the unconscious effects of child-rearing exclusively by mothers as the root of male dominance. In the more general form of her thesis, Johnson provides an analytic tool with which to look at the expression of dominance in families. She urges us to note carefully whether an adult married woman's experience of dominance in her family is attributable to her role as wife or as mother, and suggests it is the former. This distinction simultaneously draws attention to the corresponding roles for men of husband and father. It suggests that when men dominate their wives or children in families, they do so as husbands. It makes it possible to consider children as having multiple positions in families. A child is in a relationship with his mother not only as she is in the role of his mother, but also as she is in the role of "wife" in relation to the man with whom she is involved (father, stepfather, or mother's lover).

In recent years, within family therapy as within other disciplines, facing the consequences of male dominance in families has produced an explosion of awareness of family dynamics. Today, most practitioners do accept the reality of and believe in the importance of stopping intrafamilial forms of dominance, especially violence. Few people would deny the prevalence of or the disastrous consequences for women and children of wife-battering or rape, and of the emotional, physical, or sexual abuse of children.

However, there are subtler forms of dominance that take place all the time in families that may, in fact, escape notice and whose effects are also problematic. Mothers, fathers, and siblings, husbands and wives, male and female partners may all commit verbal, physical, or sexual acts of dominance in families. But I am addressing here specifically those acts of dominance that are directed toward wives, and describing the consequences for women and children contemporaneously and over generations of these acts.

I am deliberately focusing on subtle acts of dominance, for I believe that dominance exists as a continuum. I feel certain that it will not serve families well if we talk only about those forms of abuse that have crossed our collective thresholds—like husbands raping wives—and remain silent about those forms of dominance that have not received social recognition as "certifiable" forms of dominance or abuse. I know from personal and clinical experience that subtle, infrequent, nonphysical dominance can have negative, if different, effects on those who resist, submit, or observe as surely as will blatant, repetitive physical dominance.

Furthermore, as I hope this book makes clear, there are subtle forms of dominance that involve controlling the definition of reality. Dominance can assist the production of a consensus about the way things are, for instance, by controlling the definition of what is acceptable or not, what is true or false. Although the outcome of this kind of abuse is different from the outcome of physical assault, both do harm. And since dominance is often denied by those who dominate, the confusion produced by its subtler forms may be perplexing indeed.

I am not without my own confusions about these issues. To borrow from the form my children use these days to make a point humorously, it is as if, growing up, I learned: "Wives should serve their husbands. *Not*" alongside the opposite: "Wives shouldn't serve their husbands. *Not*."

In thinking about the point at which this contradiction entered my mind, I wonder whether I learned something different from each of my two roles. As my father's daughter I was encouraged to speak up, but as my mother's daughter I was discouraged from commenting on my parents' relationship. Or did my parents' expectations of me as a future wife differ from their expectations of me as a child living with a mother who was a wife? That is, as *parents* did they encourage me to believe I could and must resist domination by a husband, while as a *married couple* did they exact silence about the occasional episodes of dominance by my father with which they struggled?

I try to decipher what happened in my family: I was expected to resist domination when (not if) I became a wife but also prohibited from commenting on any episodes in which I observed my father dominate my mother. For—and this is what becomes so confusing—I may have seen my father dominate my mother, but from their perspective the domination was taking place inside their husband-wife relationship, a relationship in which I, the child, had no role, and therefore no right to comment. If I had been allowed to comment, I would have had to talk about the ways their relationship affected me, and, since I couldn't "know" this, I couldn't speak about it either. Additionally, because they didn't want their relationship to include dominance, they denied that it did. Everybody's silence was required by the denial.

This situation has left me with lingering confusions concerning what I know about life in the family I grew up in. Still, it is clear to me that I developed the idea that a woman who becomes a wife takes on a vulnerability to domination with the relationship itself. And I know for myself, from my own experience and from the clinical work that I do, that this vulnerability can be hazardous to a wife's children.

The Family Dynamics of Dominance

When I read Nina Schneider's novel, *The Woman Who Lived in a Prologue,* it set up immediate and intense resonances for me. Ariadne Arkady, Schneider's heroine, is a perfect example of a Euro-American, middle-class wife whose vulnerability affects not only herself but her children. Writing from the perspective of her seventy years, Schneider's heroine is self-consciously aware of the bargains she made and the "arrangement" within which she lived. In one of the book's many long flashbacks, she and her husband, Adam, are sitting at the table with their four children. Ariadne, the mother, is the first-person narrator:

> My first-born, my favored child, enviably free of the ordinary hopelessness that comes from learning what most desire comes to, emanated, in his young maleness, a kind of violent second presence, which in its narcissism, its inaccessibility, its aggressive masculine stance, had the allure of power.
>
>   "Gee I wish I could go . . . I wish I wish . . . Hey Mom . . ."
>
> The voice of His Highness, the Child, challenges me to feats of placation. That voice must be part of the race's survival weaponry. Built in, like the upstream drive behind a salmon's fertility, it can shoot a parent back from the adult brine to the sweet source, the amniotic waters where maternal delusions of omnipotence bathe each embryo in perfect bliss. So, to confess it plainly, I, a responsible adult, surrendered us to my son's imperious will. I blurted out, "Your wish is granted, my son. Let's all go fishing."
>
> Shock flashed through us all. Even me.
>
> The man of the house stared at me, not with pleasure. Absolom [her son] closed his eyes, lids pulsing between brows and lashes like moths still folded and damp between brown hostile twigs. Then my reward.

His lids fluttered open, pupils gone all to light turned
to me dazzled with love as if they stared into
the sun.

Adam took time to collect himself. "Your mother . . ."
I was grateful for the capsule of courtesy in which he en-
cased himself, though a look of distaste did slip through
his defenses. "Your mother seems to have declared a holiday for us all." His mouth was so compressed it flattened
and snipped off each phoneme.

The four children absorbed the drop in temperature.
Four heads bobbed from father to mother like jonquils
whipped in a fresh breeze. Absolom shivered.

I sat gaping at what had emerged from me. I reassem-
bled myself as a proper wife and mother, yet I had a
crawly suspicion that I had indulged Absolom, gained his
favor—but not for his good. I bowed my head over my
coffee cup to hide from the children's gaze. Shame
flushed through me as I bargained with the future: "Oh
Absolom, in a time of hate, recall this moment of our il-
licit joy."

Across our two coffee cups Adam and I looked at each
other and looked away. I flashed a weak, placating smile
at him. . . .

In this remarkable passage, the reader is presented with the
"rules" that govern Ariadne even as she momentarily breaks
loose from them. The passage reveals what I sensed growing up:
a wife's relationship with her husband can profoundly affect her
relationship with her children, and not, as Ariadne says, for
"good."

This young male, as his mother describes him and as we can
"observe" for ourselves, is already a person of rank and privilege,
a boy on his way to assuming the mantle of dominance that his
father wears. Ironically, he is being groomed for it as much by
his mother's "indulgence" as by his father's example.

Knowing what each of them wants, she supports the son
against the father. The terms are set: she can act on her fantasy

of omnipotence and "grant" her son his wish, or acquiesce to her husband's dominance and say nothing or "No."

It is a small enough act. Harmless on the surface. Yet it is an act of defiance. In her own "amniotic waters" of maternal omnipotence she dares to defy her husband. The effects are swift. Her son shivers; her children feel the chill that descends upon them from their mother's husband, and they, like jonquils, are "whipped."

This metaphor is not carelessly chosen. In this family, the mother's defiance will not result in physical violence to her or her children, but in other families, it is precisely such violence that is feared by mothers. Mothers who do fear violence may be more careful than Ariadne; they may be silent rather than risk the wrath of the dominant husband descending upon the should-have-been-submissive wife and her "rotten" kids.

Adam, the husband, takes control by naming the situation. He transforms, "Let's all go fishing" into "We are taking a holiday." Yet, who is taking a holiday from what? Surely Ariadne, whose "job" is the care of four children, a husband, and a household, is not taking a holiday of any sort. No, it is Adam who will be taking a holiday—one in which he will be served by a guilty wife who is already reassembling herself as a "proper wife and mother."

She knows there will be a price to pay for her moment of voice, the audacity of deciding what all of them will do. She knows, too, that she has gained her son's favor "but not for his good." Curiously, this little phrase can be read in many ways: not for his *good,* but for his detriment; not for *his* good, but for her husband's comeuppance; not for his good, but for her own need to break loose, even if for a moment, from the confining idea that her husband's wishes control her fate and the fates of her children.

This moment, brief though it may be, can be placed on a dominance continuum in which relatively minor acts of taking control, such as Adam's, fall on one end and sustained acts of terror fall on the other. Children who witness any of these acts tend to identify with the same-sex adult, though not always and not only. What is learned from these episodes will intersect with the culturally specific and family-specific messages about what it is to be a son or daughter the "right" way.

Observing Husbands and Wives

First, children learn what will be expected of them in the future by noting how adult men and adult women interact. The complexities of this education were brought home to me one day in a consultation with a couple who had been in treatment with a male therapist for about two years. They were now seeking help concerning their older son, aged twelve, who was defiant toward his mother. The question they posed was "Who needs therapy?"

The therapist described the mother to me as a woman who was comfortable with and good at taking care of others, and the father as a man who was comfortable with being taken care of. Both did backbreaking work in factories from 8:00 AM to 5:00 PM each day. The husband often worked overtime for additional money. Both came from traditional households in which fathers left home to work and later had fun with the "guys," and women stayed home taking care of the house, the children, and, frankly, their husbands.

This couple had experienced significant difficulties in their marriage as they tried to blend a new family life-style with their traditional expectations and values. Carol, the wife, had pro-tested about their arrangement first, and they shared some of their pretherapy life with me during the interview.

Carol said she had been worn out and angry constantly. She used to cry a lot in frustration, because George, her husband, could see that she was "going down the drain" but wouldn't pitch in. She said she yelled all the time at him and their two sons.

George agreed it had been "a terrible bunch of years." He said he had married a nice person and at times he felt she had turned into a monster. Therapy, he said, had made him realize that he had created the monster by his selfishness.

"What do you think you have learned in therapy that has had the most impact on you?" I asked George.

After a long pause, he replied, "You can't have two mothers."

"Say more," I responded, leaning forward in my chair.

"Well," he said, "when I was young, my mother did everything for me. She brought me breakfast in bed, and took care of me. Then when I got married, Carol did all that. Then it got to a point where she just stopped. It was like 'You can't have that anymore.' At first, I would get to her—you know, the guilt-trip thing—but then that stopped working too. It was like 'You want it? It's there. Get it yourself.' Which is right, but . . . I'd been using her, taking advantage, but I liked it. It was nice."

George's candor was disarming. I told him I thought he was sharing with us something he liked that we all like: to be mothered, to feel cared about. "The only difficulty, George, was that you wanted Carol to take care of you when she thought the two of you should be taking care of your babies together. She didn't want to take care of a . . ."

"Big baby," he finished the sentence.

It was exactly what I was going to say. Though we had been talking for only forty-five minutes or so, I felt that rapport had been quickly established and that they both could feel my respect for them, allowing me to take the liberty of confronting George with language that could have been insulting if it had been offered uncaringly.

"So, George," I said, "how do you think things might be for you if instead of a twelve-year-old son, you had a twelve-year-old daughter? Do you think you might be tempted to encourage *her* to be like a mother?"

He laughed, wiggled in his chair, and tapped his fingers on his knee. "Maybe. Probably. I think so."

It was enough time on George. I sensed that he was ready for Carol to answer the same question. "What do you think you learned in therapy, Carol?" I asked.

"I learned to sit on my hands," she replied emphatically. "I used to go through a room and automatically pick up and straighten things out, and now I don't. I used to feel bad if I didn't, but I don't now."

From this comment, she led directly into the current problem. Their oldest boy refused to do what she asked of him. By making deals with him—she would do this, if he would do that—she could get situational compliance, but in general he refused to do what was asked of him without a struggle.

"If I ask him to do something, he says 'No.' I have to nag or confront him before he will do what I say. It has to be a fight. I really can't figure out what he's thinking."

Hoping to broaden the context within which we might understand her son's behavior, I asked what he observed at home. "Does he see other people do what they are asked or told to do?"

Carol looked over at George, and smiled wryly. "Don't look at me," George told her.

"George is the type," Carol went on, "that if I ask him, he'll do anything, but he won't see to do it. I have to walk into the room and then say to do something for him to notice what needs to be done. The little one will do what we ask."

"And Carol will," George chimed in.

George's version of his response to requests from Carol was quite different from hers. In his version, he did not respond positively. "I tell her over and over, 'You say something to me in front of the kids; don't do that! You're making trouble.' They see me and they say, 'Why do I have to do it if Dad doesn't? She should take me aside and tell me. Not tell me in front of the boys."

"To me it seems like he should set an example for them," replied Carol. "But he thinks they should listen to him and do what he says, not what he does."

George believes he should do more of the work at home. Still, he wants to do it in a way that preserves the appearance of his dominance over his wife and children. He wants his children to obey him, even if *his* behavior contradicts what he tells them to do. And he does not want his children to see that he does what his wife tells him to do.

What messages are his sons getting? They are learning that husbands dominate (or want to dominate, or believe they should dominate) wives. They are learning that husbands can do this verbally and nonverbally, but always their efforts are aimed at controlling the definition of the situation. Sites for domination of this sort may include the wife's body itself, her belongings, her activities, and her relationships, including those with her children.

Domination of the Wife's Body

Increasingly, children are witnessing violent acts toward their mothers, whether by their fathers or by men with whom their mothers are involved. There is little doubt about the traumatizing potential of witnessing such acts for children and of being so victimized for the mother. Violence inflicted on a woman's body causes pain, wounds, and terror; it also erodes her sense of mastery over her body. With repeated violation, her body can seem to belong to the person who is abusing it.

Though this may seem odd, during my cancer treatment, I had experiences with my health-care providers in which I came to feel that my body was not my own. I repeatedly encountered a view of my breasts that disconfirmed my own. I hated those times, and I suspect that one of the reasons I did was that they made me feel like a "wife."

After my diagnosis, I was given a choice: medically, my risks of survival would be equal whether I chose mastectomy or lumpectomy with radiation. Having no reason to doubt the data, no reason to challenge the statistics, I moved on to ask the kinds of questions the answers to which would help me make my choice. (Not thinking of having more children, I didn't ask whether lumpectomy with radiation would allow me to nurse, though clearly mastectomy would not have.) I asked, "What will my breast feel like?"

The answers were unnerving. From men and women alike, nurses and doctors, the answer was the same: "Depending on your skin's response to the radiation, it will be coarse or not, feel the same or harder." Each person was responding with the answer to a question I had not asked, "What will my breast feel like to someone's (my husband's, my) touch?" But that question, at that moment, was far from my mind.

I wanted to know, as the subject of my own desire, not the object of my husband's desire, or anyone else's, what my breast would feel like to me; what sensations I would still experience; what delicate connections between the brain, the breast, and the genitals would be snapped by the well-meaning, but brutal, burning X rays? Nobody, but nobody, understood my question. It turned out, later, that nobody *could* answer it.

I asked my primary radiotherapist, "What will my breast feel like?"

"I can't answer that," he replied. "We don't know the answer."

"Because you've never asked?"

"That's right," he said. "We don't ask."

I don't know what he thought he was revealing when he said, "We don't ask." I suspect that he thought he was stating a simple case: How would one interpret data that would be so complex in this context? How could one sort out the psychological from the physiological effects of radiation? But I think he was revealing much more, if not particularly about himself. In fact, I found him and most of my health-care providers free from any sexist attitudes toward me that would have made me feel uncomfortable and alienated. Nonetheless, the situation revealed a prejudice about breasts that is common in our culture: breasts do not belong only to the woman; they belong also to the people who desire them.

I had trouble complaining about this attitude, because I appreciated how fortunate I was to have gotten cancer after the women who came before me had worked so hard on other issues. That is, my doctors, educated by these women, took as axiomatic that breast surgery evokes feelings of grief, associated with the loss of the breast as a loved body part, and they knew that it is important, not frivolous, to try to achieve as good a cosmetic result as possible. Perhaps they learned these lessons so well that they had trouble hearing from a patient whose issues

veered slightly from the path. My concern was sensation and
loss, not cosmesis and loss.

Each time a doctor examined my breasts—thirty times? a
hundred?—and told me how they looked, I got angry. I felt that
the doctor, man or woman, was revealing that women are seen
as objects for the pleasure of men; that women's breasts, which
allow such sweet pleasure sucked by whomever they choose, are
objects of male domination even when they have cancer and
need care. I was in the thrall of a dominant perspective on
breasts, which was overriding my particular experience and erasing my efforts to define it. My question "What will I feel?" was
my effort to define the nature of my experience, and the absence
of any information on that subject compellingly signaled that my
concerns were marginalized by a dominant way of thinking
about breasts. To me, it was an aspect of how, I believe, many
people think about wives and women. Their bodies are not entirely their own.

Training Boys/Training Girls

A husband may dominate his wife through attempting to
control her body ("You are too fat"; "You are too thin"; "I want
sex now"), or through control of her activities ("I can't be home
to watch the kids tonight, so you can't go out with your
friends"), or through control of her relationship with her children. Freud's Oedipal theory can be read as an example of just
such an instance of a husband dominating his wife by controlling her relationship to her son. According to this view, the Oedipal theory records a husband's insistence that his wife distance
herself from her son so that the young male child will not feel
dominated by a woman. Freud believed that the father interrupts
the son's attachment to his mother by threatening the son's masculinity. In an intriguing interpretation of the Oedipus complex,
Miriam M. Johnson raises two interesting paired questions: Why
doesn't the son's heterosexual attachment to his mother ensure
his masculinity? Why must the boy relinquish this love? Her
answer is that it is not the "right" kind of heterosexual love, for

it is a love in which the mother, by virtue of her generation, is dominant over her son. The boy must relinquish the mother not because she is an improper love choice, but because he cannot be dominant over her.

Johnson's theory permits us to distinguish who redirects the son's love: It is not the boy's father; rather, it is the mother's husband. At the same time, the father, that is, the wife's husband, offers the son identification with him in place of the intense relationship with the mother. The father, often with the enthusiastic cooperation of the mother, offers to help the son become a little man. To accomplish this goal, the father may insist that his wife diminish her mothering of the boy. "Don't make a sissy out of him" is a common refrain of fathers.

I believe that a boy suffers terribly from the loss of maternal solicitude and care at this point. What's more, a son may witness his father benefiting from his wife's mothering and feel further deprived. The apparent contradiction is resolvable when we consider that the father encourages the son to renounce his relationship to his mother until he is old enough to be the dominant partner in a relationship with a woman, while the father, who is the dominant partner with his wife, is free to enjoy her motherliness.

In some respects, what the father offers the son at this time is training in domination. George's behavior in his family can be understood from this perspective. However, it simultaneously creates dilemmas for George. Though he does not want his son to defy his mother, neither does he want his son to be dominated by his wife, for this threatens the "proper" relationship between men and women. Not surprisingly, George and Carol were in a quandary about who needs therapy. At one point in the interview, quite seriously, I proposed that "the culture" needs therapy.

Clearly, not all cultures are the same, but in George and Carol's culture male dominance is the norm. This plays out directly with their sons, and George acknowledges that it would probably be a factor if he had a daughter. If George had had a daughter, he acknowledged, he might have been tempted to train her to mother him, which he could accomplish by encouraging her to be a daddy's girl, or little wife. By encouraging his daughter to serve him, through rewarding her for her favors, a father can receive more "mothering" while maintaining his position of dominance.

I was not a typical 1950s daddy's girl. I enjoyed a relationship with my father so free of what I saw all around me that I was convinced that my parents' treatment of me meant that my father had wanted a boy. Many details signaled my difference from other daughters, coded as they were as not "daddy's girlish." At five, I threw a fit when my best friend showed up for a trip to New York with my father and me in a frilly pink dress puffed out by a crinoline. My mother had dressed me in tailored plaid. My friend wore black Mary Jane's, whereas I had on brown oxfords. She was dressed for Daddy, and I could now see that I wasn't.

At seven, I worked with my father in the garden and I remember the feeling of daring and sharing that came with us both stripped to the waist and heaving rocks out of the newly spaded earth. At ten, we took long walks in the woods, enjoying the pleasure of each other's company. By sixteen, my father staged debates with me, honing my abilities to sustain an argument. He treated me with respect and interest; I was not groomed to serve. In this, I was not taught to be a wife. However, I did learn habits of silence in the face of his domination of my mother that could easily have rolled out into place had my marriage taken a different direction.

Miranda is not being groomed to serve. At eleven, Miranda told me that she was not like many of the other girls. "They flirt, Mom. They look like girls in the movies; they puff themselves up and slide around the boys. I'm not interested in boys that way yet." I haven't the heart to tell her that she may never be interested "that way." For her father and I are not grooming her to be a girl like that. She and Hilary catch turtles together; he teaches her physics; they watch *The Marriage of Figaro* and play French horns together. They wrestle a lot. It's hard for me to imagine where she will learn to be a wife, although she has two parents from whom she can learn to be a loving partner.

In the matter of silence, what we are teaching her is harder to evaluate. She appears to feel free to talk about all that transpires, but then, could I ever discover what she doesn't let herself know she knows? If she does feel silenced, her silence would have to fall inside a blind spot, which, by definition, I cannot perceive. I can only hope that Hilary and I have made it clear enough that we respect respectful challenges. In fact, I would say that making that clear is one of our most important jobs. It is a way that we can communicate that our children, too, are part of a loving partnership with us. And that, I believe, is the solution to George's dilemma. Before I elaborate, though, there is more to be said about the family dynamics of dominance in regard to wives.

The Family Dynamics of Abusive Dominance

As I have mentioned, dominance exists as a continuum. When dominance is abusive, when dominance engenders terror and helplessness, trauma can happen. Then, into the mix of male-female relations, couple and parental ones both, additional messages are transmitted and behaviors learned. In the last decade, clinicians and researchers have identified ways in which witnessing violence can disrupt normal developmental trajectories and produce short-term coping strategies that have devastating long-term consequences.

By conservative estimates, each year in the United States thousands of children witness extreme acts of violence involving at least one parent. Wife battering and rape are two of the most common acts of violence children witness. Although experts have different opinions as to the specific effects that witnessing violence has on later adult behavior, none of them believes that the impact is neutral or benign.

As a family therapist, I am impressed by the long reach into future generations that violence in one generation can have many decades hence. Coming from a European Jewish household, I find it ironic that my ability to trace my own family's history of violence back to the shtetls in which my great-grand-parents lived has been forever foreclosed by the epic acts of traumatizing domination—the pogroms and the Holocaust—that my family, like other Jewish families, suffered. My maternal grandfather, who was traumatized repeatedly in his childhood, both within his family and as a Jew in his community, was unable to talk about his parents beyond a few noncommunicative words. Like many other victims of violence, he would not, perhaps could not, speak about many of the events he recalled.

However, his response to the violence that he saw, the terror and helplessness he felt, seems to have been different from the response of his daughter to the violence she witnessed. He grew up to be a man with a violent temper, which he expressed verbally to his wife and daughter; his daughter, having witnessed these marital battles, subsequently never once yelled at a family member. She was affected in very particular ways by what she had witnessed, not the least of which was her maintenance of silence regarding the violence she saw.

My mother's ability to protect herself from dominant moves in some contexts was seriously hampered, I think, because she had difficulty mobilizing anger on her own behalf. A few years before she died, she hauntingly described her anger as buried deep within herself, in a coffin. "I cannot get to it if my life depends on it."

Historically, as I understand it, my mother was terrified of her father's temper. She witnessed it when very young, during her parents' few years in San Francisco trying to make a go of the delicatessen venture, unbuffered by the comfort and consolation of kin, who were all back in Brooklyn. By the time her mother left her father, and mother and daughter took that long train ride across the continent, my mother had developed the idea, as so many children who witness wife battering do, that her parents' fighting was her fault. She vowed to be a better little girl, which meant to her that she should never show anger. Alas, in this, as in so many other lifetime goals, she succeeded brilliantly.

Where anger was not appropriate, her parenting skills were admirable. Where anger might be natural, her behavior was sometimes, but not always, off. One episode is particularly salient to me, for through this event, I can observe the linkage among my grandfather, my mother, myself, and my daughter around the issue of abusive dominance. On the surface it is a story about hair, but, underneath, it is a story about violation and protest, and the complicated ways in which we teach children, and children learn, to protect themselves against encroachments. In this story, none of the family members commits an act that would rate as abusive by most people, and yet it seems to me necessary to know about the dynamics of traumatic abuse to understand this tale fully.

When I was twelve, my mother and I were shopping while my sister, Jan, got a haircut at a department store in Manhattan. We were dressed for town, with long coats and short white gloves. At the appointed hour, my mother sent me into the hair salon to let my sister know that we were in the waiting area. I walked up to Jan's chair, bent over to tell her, and the hairdresser, a dark-haired man in his thirties, leaned toward me with his shears and snipped my right braid off at the root. Shocked, I whirled around to face him. I remember seeing him wave the scissors and I remember seeing his mouth move as if it were uttering syllables, but I have no memory of what he was saying. I ran from the room to my mother and collapsed sobbing into her arms.

She was very calm. Implacably so, I would say. She took me by the hand and led me to his chair. She asked him if he had finished my sister's haircut. I have no idea what he replied. She then told me to sit in the chair and told him to cut off the other braid so that at least my hair would be even. She looked like an ice queen — erect, still, stern. I allowed him to chop off the other braid. We did not take them home.

My mother took me by the hand, walked over to the cashier, paid for my sister's haircut, and, with a voice like a stretched filament, told the woman that of course she would not pay for mine. We took the elevator to another floor, where she bought a scarf to cover my shorn head. Still gripping my hand, she led us to the subway to my father's office. It was rush hour, and we three were squeezed together on the seats of the train. With my shorn and babushkaed head, I had only one association, which I felt too ashamed to share. How could I possibly equate the misery I felt with the suffering of my Jewish relatives who had ridden to their deaths? But I did.

My mother, who had been hauled off by the police in front of her children to testify to the House Un-American Activities Committee during the 1950s, and gave no names, though her children and husband were threatened, was a brave woman. She never lacked courage. But in a New York department store, in a cloth coat and white gloves, she did not get angry. Not only did I see her restrain her anger, but she made me sit in the chair to have the other braid cut off. Though her intention was to force this man to correct his mistake, from my perspective she failed to protect me from further violation. Had she been unconflicted about her own anger toward angry men, I feel confident that she would have chosen a different means of redress. I can no more imagine letting a child of mine back into the hands of a demented hairdresser than I can imagine flying to the moon. But then, this kind of out-of-control angry man isn't familiar and frightening to me, since I did not grow up with one. When I *am* confused and vulnerable, though, I, like my mother, inadvertently participate in my children's violation as well. Not surprisingly, I am vulnerable in regard to hair.

When I found out I would need chemotherapy, one side effect of which can be loss of hair, I went to be fitted for a wig. My waist-length hair was too long to fit one. I had to make the preemptive decision to cut my hair so that, if I lost it, I would have a wig immediately available. Miranda, who had long hair in defiance of her classmates' pressure to cut it off and be "cool," was devastated by my choice, but understanding. She chose to go with me for my haircut, to be my witness and, as it turned out, to save every scrap of hair. I promised her I would grow it back as soon as I could, but I have not. I refuse ever to cut long hair again. I won't let my hair grow long, because I fear that I may have to cut it again. What does cutting long hair mean to me? Not just the loss of my hair, not just the fear of death, but the loss of protection against, and participation in, my own violation.

How can I share these meanings with Miranda, all of which I suspect she could understand, since the cornerstone of my position rests on the idea that I might have to cut my hair again? How can I tell my daughter, who believes I am cured, that I fear I might not be? How can I protect her from worry where I am confused and vulnerable? Because I do not know the answers to these questions, this is a conversation we do not have.

Instead, we have a different talk. Periodically she tells me that I have betrayed her: "You promised me you would grow back your hair and you haven't. I will never forgive you for this." Her anger is clear and direct. My implacability in response, so alien to our relationship, is clear, direct, and fundamentally mystifying. I tell her, "I'm sorry. I didn't know how I was going to feel."

I am defining what we will and will not speak about, and in doing so, though I have my reasons, I dominate her. I am also doing exactly what I need to do. I could say to her, "I don't want to talk to you about this, and our relationship has to have enough flexibility to include each of us wanting privacy at some time," but I don't say that. I don't want to talk about it at all. She cannot know what I don't want to tell her, but she can feel that I am withholding something crucial from her. I could not know what my mother did not want to tell me. Or perhaps my mother didn't know that the angry man waving the scissors reminded her of her father shouting at her mother, in a scene all too familiar and frightening to her. But I absorbed, as I am sure Miranda is doing, lessons she didn't want me to learn. I learned that women are afraid of men; that men can commit senseless acts of violence and not be punished for it. I learned that women may be afraid to hold men accountable, or be unable to do so. I cannot know with any certainty what Miranda is learning. But one thing is clear. She must "know" that the relationship of mutuality that we both so clearly cherish is more mine than hers to control. At the heart of any situations of domination, even in ones that are relatively benign, is just such an asymmetry. Part of what drives the intergenerational transmission of abuse and violation is the helplessness that follows in the wake of such asymmetry of control.

Exit-Voice Dilemmas

If dominance in families becomes untenable, wives often leave husbands. When there are children, however, they may believe that their mothers are leaving their fathers. They may fail to distinguish that the man whom their mother can no longer tolerate is her husband, not their father. Ironically, it is often when men become fathers and women become mothers that dominance in marriage, as expressed, for instance, in wife battering, begins or accelerates. In fact, studies have shown that pregnancy is a particularly vulnerable time for women in relation to men's violence.

The decision to leave a marriage is often difficult for wives, but these same women may find it even harder to consider breaking up their families. Again, their two family roles—wife and mother—may pull them in different directions. Thinking as mothers, wives may let economic and custody concerns take precedence over issues of safety. The tension is often unbearably painful, the choices dreadful. During this time of agonizing, it is almost certain that a woman will be unable to talk to her husband about her dilemma. Marriages that are in crisis are ones in which people have been unable to listen well to each other for a very long time, if they ever did.

Susan Moller Okin, a political scientist, has an interesting perspective on the dilemmas women face in leaving a marriage. She applies an economist's theory to the situation of marriage, speculating that the development of voice proceeds most effectively when exit is possible but not too attractive. That is, people will most often talk about—voice—their thoughts and feelings about their marriages, presumably hoping that speaking will lead to improvements, when they are clear that they can exit—leave their marriages—but would prefer to stay.

In my own life, this formulation rings true. Until I became sick, I believed that exit was always a possibility for me in my marriage. Economically, I felt certain that I would be able to support myself and the children alone if I had to do so. Nor did I ever worry that Hilary would be violent to me were I to consider leaving—a risk for many wives—or distant from the children in consequence. The possibility of exit, though never appealing, was inextricably related to my ability to stay in voice in my relationship.

After treatment, by contrast, I felt profoundly dependent on Hilary. Emotionally exhausted, wracked by terror, physically spent, I could not imagine surviving without his steady, lovingkindness. Psychologically, exit no longer felt like an option. Corresponding to that perception, I stopped speaking to him about our marriage. I, who had always been interested in "working on our issues," went silent about them. More important, I stopped observing the instances of conflict that our relationship usually piled up in a week or month—in effect, losing my ability to know what I knew. Voice, which I had always thought of as a stable characteristic of mine with my husband, I learned was dependent on my context.

Okin's book looks at the economic and legal context of marriage as related to exit and voice. She finds that marriage itself makes women vulnerable. Marriage does so by setting up girls to believe that they will be the primary caretakers of children, and that "in fulfilling this role they will need to try to attract and to keep the economic support of a man, to whose work life they will be expected to give priority. They are rendered vulnerable by the actual division of labor within almost all current marriages. They are disadvantaged at work by the fact that the world of wage work, including the professions, is still largely structured around the assumption that 'workers' have wives at home. They are rendered far more vulnerable if they become the primary caretakers of children, and their vulnerability peaks if their marriage dissolves and they become single parents."

Okin analyzes how various circumstances create economic dependencies for mothers on their husbands. These vulnerabilities have important effects during marriage (and may have catastrophic effects for women and children after marriages dissolve). Many a mother, looking around her at the plight of mothers and children she knows, has silenced her voice or found herself with nothing to say, but is left with a pervasive malaise that insidiously and insistently grinds away at her, at her husband, and at her children.

If a mother lets herself know fully what she knows to be so about her marriage—when there isn't enough love, or comfort, or commitment, or mutuality to make the trade-offs worthwhile—then she must assess the impact of the dissolution of the marriage not only on herself but also on her children. Okin's analysis is clear. After divorce, mothers and children are severely disadvantaged by gender-blind legal practices that misconstrue the actual situation in contemporary marriage and operate to sustain the same level of vulnerability after marriage that the woman sustained in anticipation of and during marriage. The picture is bleak.

Ironically, it is precisely in attempting to treat men and women as equals at the end of marriage that inequality is perpetuated. I would add that it is in attempting to treat the father/ husband roles as comparable to the mother/wife roles that a flawed analysis occurs. Most commonly, divorce for women and children means a loss of income, though the extent of the drop and the duration are matters of dispute. Estimates place the loss of income as between 33% and 73%. Despite these grim economic prospects, many wives leave their husbands. Not surprisingly, wives are more likely to leave husbands if they have a means of supporting themselves and their children. Also, wives are more likely to leave husbands if they believe that their husbands will not challenge them for custody of their children. Concern about losing their children is yet another context that influences exit-voice.

In *Mothers on Trial*, Phyllis Chesler passionately describes the fate of mothers who exit marriages and then face the threat or actual loss of their children. One consequence of some modern divorces is that husbands sue mothers for custody of children even when they have not been the primary parent to the child. Husbands sue mothers for custody for a variety of reasons, the elucidation of which, Chesler believes, reveals the "tip of a custodial iceberg" showing how "men, individually and collectively, can either subsidize a woman's motherhood—or can prevent, regulate, profit from, or destroy a woman's motherhood." According to Chesler, custody battles reveal patterns of male domination between women and their heterosexual partners.

Chesler's central thesis is that the criteria for the "good-enough" mother and the "good-enough" father are dramatically different, depending as they do on social constructions of mothering and fathering. Her data suggest that the criteria for being a good-enough mother are perilously fused with those a husband might use for a good-enough wife. As Chesler describes it, not-good-enough mothers have committed three sorts of "crimes" that lead to custodial victimization by their husbands: the mother is sexual with a man outside the marriage; she is "uppity," by which Chesler means she worked outside the home, wanted a divorce, or wanted to move; and/or she is a lesbian. Put differently, mothers are penalized for failing to submit to husbands.

In a moving personal story written under the pseudonym Anna Demeter, one mother has recorded her experience of uncoupling from a cruel and tyrannical husband, for which she nearly paid with the loss of her life and her children. A tale of awesome courage and compassion, her book, *Legal Kidnaping,* also chronicles a path from silence to voice. It opens with an immediacy that is sustained throughout: "I thought I had to make a gesture of suicide to resolve the problem of my marriage. The 'problem' of my marriage was the marriage itself. In nineteen years of a mostly traditional marriage, contracted in the spirit of the 1950s, I had been chronically terrified of Michael's rage; most of all I was terrified of the rage I thought he would turn on me if I said I did not want to live with him any longer. From the beginning I had felt that my legal alliance with him was irrevocable: when I became his wife I became a possession—one of his most valued—and as the possession of a rageful man I did not feel that divorce was a possible option for me."

On the other hand, conditions with Michael were unbearable. Finally she made a suicide gesture, thinking that if she died she would avoid the awful responsibility of a divorce, and if she lived, she would take it as a sign that she should proceed. After the attempt, which she survived, she asked Michael for a divorce; his response followed shortly. He kidnapped their two youngest children, and Anna lived through the harrowing months of their absence, the necessity of maintaining a home and earning a living for her other children, and the failures of the legal system to help her recover her children from their father, a legal kidnapper.

Though the law is different now, at the time her book was written, 1977, there was only one state in which parental kidnapping was a felony. As Anna Demeter worked with detectivelike skill to recover her children, she simultaneously uncovered and exposed the social constructions of mother-right, father-right, and child-right that had such critical and devastating consequences for her family's life.

Legal Kidnaping makes explicit the connections between male dominance and its impact, not just on mothers' lives, but on children's as well. The book traces one family's efforts to break free of relations of dominance to ones of intimate collaboration. One of Anna's children, at the end of the book, when her siblings have come home and they are starting the saga of visitations to their father, says: "Maybe when we go visit Dad, if we keep him company, he will lose his violence."

Forming Loving Partnerships

Anna Demeter's wise young daughter is speaking about a crucial change that must take place on the most intimate, as well as on the community, national, and global level. Somehow, relations characterized by dominance must be transformed to ones of mutuality and collaboration. It is in this spirit that I have told Hilary that I cannot be his wife, though I am happy to be his loving partner.

Years ago, when many people good-humoredly talked about wanting a wife, I never thought it funny. Would I joke about wanting a slave? In my mind, no one should have, or be, a wife, if by wife they mean what I mean—a person who is not equal to her adult partner. Yet I know the deep satisfactions that come from caring for and being cared for by another when the relationship is one of mutual love, trust, and respect. I do think that life is easier and more gratifying if men and women have loving partners.

Some women will choose men as the loving partners with whom to share their lives and raise children. For heterosexual couples, however, working out equal parenting arrangements will not, I fear, as some feminist theorists have proposed, solve the problems of male dominance. For if husbands dominate wives *while* sharing child-care equally, patterns of dominance will persist, not disappear. Instead, husbands' domination must change. This will happen when male dominance becomes unacceptable at every level, from the trivial to the great.

In order for dominance to become unacceptable, people will have to be able to perceive and comment on it. Inside the family, we will have to help each other recognize and resist subtle forms of dominance as well as more blatant ones. Outside the family, in our surroundings, we will also, as a nation, have to learn to identify as domination and violence that which not all of us currently do.

Just as for centuries what existed as violence within the family did not "count," what exists as violence for millions of Americans does not officially count either. For instance, we need to count as violence maintaining families below the poverty level; failing to build affordable housing; not attempting to provide jobs to all citizens; and inequitable funding of education.

From the perspective of the wider context of societal violence, raising issues about the dynamics of dominance within marriage, as I do, may seem less important than whether, because of extrafamilial dominance, marriage can be a choice at all. In a recent

"Hers" column in the *New York Times Magazine,* an African-American mother and professor of journalism, Patricia Raybon, writes about the "promise" of marriage stolen by American racism from young African-American men and women. The piece affirms marriage and reserves its bitterness for a society that is killing African-American men. Throughout, the implicit comparison to marriage is the absence of that choice. In particular, Raybon grieves that her daughter, like other young African-American women, is denied the same chance for romance and marriage as European-American females her age have and African-American women had years ago. The young African-American woman, she writes, who is waiting to meet a potential African-American male partner, finds that the "boys are all gone. Far too many of them anyway." Gone to danger, gone to drugs, gone to frustration, gone to jail. America is abandoning and destroying young men of color, and blaming it on their own violence toward each other.

Raybon asserts that the framework of black-on-black violence is an audacious distortion. Black-on-black violence may be occurring in urban areas at alarming rates, but what is the context within which this violence is taking place? The point here, as it is inside the family, is the same: What will we allow to count; who will decide; how will those decisions be enforced; and what will the consequences be? I believe that we are beginning as a nation to grapple with the problems of "domestic violence," by which we mean the violence *inside* homes. We need to grapple as well with the violence that *surrounds* homes. We need to allow more to count as violence, so that we can work for change. Ultimately, the solution to both kinds of violence is an unprecedented level of loving partnership, spanning marital, community, cultural, ideological, national, religious, and race relations.

Inside families, some women choose other women with whom to have loving partnerships, women who may be lovers, sisters, mothers, friends, or other kin. Depending on a wide variety of circumstances, some women are disinclined to be wives, either at all or again. For some women, not being a wife is a distinctly different choice from not being a mother. These women may want to take their chances that the issues of emotional or physical dominance that certainly do exist between women will play out differently, and less problematically, in their family arrangements.

The legacy of family arrangements in which male dominance has been a part creates sons and daughters who enter their own chosen families handicapped. Sons become fathers in families of their own in which they turn to wives for the mothering they lost too early. Daughters become mothers in families of their own in which they want their husbands to be good fathers. These former-daughter mothers turn to former-son husbands and find men who long for good fathers as much as they do.

As I have thought about the layers of ideas I have about wives, I have come right up against my thinking about fathers. What did I learn about fathers when I was growing up? What did I understand about how families form and why they appear as they do? How has what I learned as a child fit with my professional work as a family therapist? I turn next to exploring my ideas about fathers, noting as I do that my ideas and feelings about fathers intersect with the emerging national dialogue about absent fathers.

SEVEN

If Fathers Are Going to Be Important . . .

Valuing Fathers/Blaming Mothers . . . Again

Most of my memories of my first four years are visual and tactile. As if they were a silent movie, rarely do I hear sounds or words. I remember my father from those long-ago mornings. In one memory, my father and sister and I are in the kitchen. I am squirming—which I feel, as if I am inside my body, and also see, as if my memory has stationed a camera at the edge of the kitchen door. My sister, who is four years older, is sitting peacefully at the table. I am positioned with my back to the one small window, looking at her, but craning my neck to see my father.

He is making us breakfast. I see him at the stove, with the large black skillet that traveled with us from place to place when we moved. I feel the moment that my body transfixes into stillness as it notices a fried egg floating through the air. A spatula is rising toward it. The round orb miraculously lands inside the hard black pan; the egg will be coming to me, coming to Jan.

Next, as if memory were a comic strip, three frames to a story, I am on the street with my father. We have dropped off Jan at her school. I feel my hand in his. It is warm there. My arm is reaching up, but my father is bearing the weight. The image in focus is my arm, our hands, and a patch of grey pavement.

The third frame. We are in the black wrought-iron-lace cage of an elevator, slowing ascending to my nursery school. I am looking up at my father and through the open grillwork. I am hopping with excitement. Another day at school. I have recorded no kiss and no good-bye. This picture sums up the routine of my morning's comfort and pleasure with Jan and with my father. My mother is at work already.

The experiences inscribed in that memory left other traces. They led me to expect that a father could do what a mother often does: provide safety, comfort, playfulness, nurturance, and financial resources. Along with other experiences, these expectations have made me believe that fathers can make a positive difference in their children's lives—that fathers are important to families.

On the surface, the current political rhetoric about fathers, its decrying of those families in which fathers are absent, appears to be about the importance of fathers to families. I wish that this were so, but I fear that it is not. If it were so, it would signal a shift of epic proportions in the conceptualization of the family. It would mean that mothers are no longer viewed as solely or principally responsible for family life, because fathers are viewed as connected as fundamentally to family as they are to the workplace, and as fundamentally connected to families as are mothers.

I am skeptical though. I fear that the new rhetoric merely masks the ages-old "blame-mothers" thinking and obscures both psychological and political truths about contemporary family life. I worry not because I think fathers are unimportant, but because I think they are so important that I wish attention were being drawn to this issue clearly, both conceptually and politically. I fear that as the inevitable critique of the absent-father rhetoric is made, as I will do in the pages that follow, we may appear to diminish the importance of fathers, when in fact we desperately need to make the case for creating conditions that allow fathers to be as competent as mothers. It is adequacy, not just absence, we desperately need to address.

In a speech in June 1992, then Vice-President Dan Quayle made the Bush and former Reagan Administrations' position on traditional family values vividly clear. He told a convention of Southern Baptists in Indianapolis that "the cultural elites respect neither tradition nor standards. They believe that moral truths are relative and all lifestyles are equal. They seem to think the family is an arbitrary arrangement of people who decide to live under the same roof, that fathers are dispensable and that parents need not be married or even of the opposite sexes. They are wrong."

In this statement, Quayle throws down the gauntlet, implying that there is one right American family: a family headed by a father, with a mother and their children. His rhetoric seems tricky to me, since I agree that fathers are important and that all life-styles are not equal. Yet the life-style to which I object is one in which fathers dominate their families, using violence or intimidation. I do believe that no father is better than a violent father, and that other competent adults, living harmoniously, can parent better than an incompetent father.

I disagree also with Quayle's assessment of who is on the front lines of change in families. He blames the new family forms—what sociologist Judith Stacey has called the postmodern family—on the "cultural elites." In doing so, he misses the point that sociologists have been documenting for years. As Stacey writes: "White, middle-class families, I have come to believe, are less the innovators than the propagandists and principal beneficiaries of contemporary family change. African-American women and white, working-class women"—not the cultural elites, as Quayle would have us believe—"have been the genuine postmodern family pioneers, even though they also suffer most from its most negative effects."

A current variety of political rhetoric also mythologizes conditions in the "traditional" family, simplifying complex family dynamic processes. Although the emphasis on fathers suits a certain conservative political agenda, it intersects with already-formed cultural tales about absent fathers. Classic texts (the stories of Odysseus, Oedipus, Hamlet), the mental-health community, and the recent Men's Movement have all been concerned with absent fathers.

Implicit in these tales of the absent father are several assumptions that I believe must be challenged. First, they suggest that an absent father is truly absent, when in fact, he may be physically but not psychologically so. Second, they presume that if father absence causes problems, father presence prevents them. Third, they assume that a two-parent family is preferable to a single-mother family, and that the second parent should be male. All of these assumptions grossly simplify complex matters that I believe deserve more serious attention.

The recent interest in absent fathers is highly politically charged. I fear that it has become shorthand for or an alternative path to blaming mothers, this time single mothers. In decrying absent fathers, I hear an implicit backhanded attack on single women, as if they are single because they have had the audacity to choose to "go it alone" without a man.

I find the subtext of blaming mothers particularly disturbing, for, as a therapist, I take as axiomatic the idea that people cannot change when their behavior is negatively connoted. The issue of making room for fathers in families is critically important. To couple an appeal for fathers with an attack on mothers is, to my mind, making an argument in such a way that you jeopardize the reception of the message.

Father Absence/Father Presence

Take the matter of whether fathers are absent or not. Though my father was always present for me, our family started as a father-absent one. My sister was born in April of 1943. Ten weeks later, my father shipped out with the Navy. After a very brief maternity leave, my mother returned to her job on the newspaper, leaving my sister with a pieced-together tapestry of childcare, including paid baby-sitters and unpaid relatives. Perhaps because my mother wanted to include my father in his daughter's development as much as she could, or perhaps because Jan was their first child, there is an extensive pictorial record of my sister's first few years.

There are also many tales. My mother used to tell the story of my sister running up to any sailor on the street and yelling "Daddy," mortifying my mother even though she quite understood Jan's reasons. My sister's total enthusiasm for these visual reminders of her father stood in stark contrast, as my mother's narrative of this time went, with her actual response to her real father when he returned from the war in late December of 1945. A cautious Jan was two years and eight months old when he returned.

As my mother explained it to me, the advice that mothers in her situation were given was to do everything possible to hasten the reintegration of their husbands into the fabric of daily life. My mother did not leave her job, as so many women did to make room for the GIs, but she did create a space for my father to enter the family and become a participatory dad. In fact, in later years, it was my mother's belief that she had been too scrupulous about stepping aside so that my father and Jan could "get to know each other." Inadvertently, she feared, she might have disrupted my sister's primary relationship with her.

Why would she have done that? My answer is a simple one. She feared that the years of my father's absence might have harmed my sister, and that she needed to do all she could to integrate him into family life. She never considered that my father had never *not* been a part of his new family. All the talk was about men's physical absence, and no one discussed how some families had managed to keep fathers, brothers, sons, and husbands psychologically present. Yet that approach might have fit the facts of their lives better. My mother not only kept my father informed by daily letters and regular photographs, but she told my sister stories of her father that surely made him a vivid character for her. Too, my father wrote home every day. Though our family would obviously have been different had my father been there, calling him absent denies the ways he was meaningfully present in my mother's and sister's lives.

My father and Jan did develop a strong affection and alliance. Not infrequently their alliance excluded others, particularly my mother. My mother, believing it only right that my father make up for lost time, rarely insisted that they form a trio. So powerful was her idea of restitution, so concerned was she about what the latent impact on both Jan and my father might be of his absence, so unable to look at what the aftermath of these arrangements might be on her, that she never protested the asymmetric shape the family was taking. And neither, of course, did they. When she became pregnant with me, four months after my father came home, she was sure that balance would be restored. My father had Jan and she would have me.

In later years, I shared stories with younger siblings whose older siblings, like mine, had started off life in a father-absent, single-mother home, becoming a two-parent family later. These families seemed to share certain characteristics with mine. These families, too, seemed to retain the double configuration of father-absent/father-present dynamics.

One anecdote from when I was four and my sister was eight perfectly evokes the feeling of these early childhood years for me, although the event was not representative of our family life. Rather, it was what is called in statistics an outlier, an incident found on the extreme of my family's range, expressing one unlikely, but disturbing, outcome of our way of being together. Unlike so many family stories, this is one that we all used to tell later, whenever something would remind us of the event. It is surely one of the most dramatic family moments the four of us ever shared.

One day, soon after my mother had stopped her job as a reporter and was trying to be a housewife, she made a pie. It was a big, fluffy, lemon-meringue and the very first pie she had ever baked. My sister and I were beside ourselves with excitement all afternoon, anticipating the glorious moment when my mother would bring in the pie after dinner and, to my father's astonished face, yell: "Surprise!" The moment came and it was memorable. My duly-impressed father marveled at my mother's creation.

Next—and there are different versions of this moment—my sister turned to my father and said, "Do you dare me to throw this pie in your face?" to which he replied, "Yes!" My sister did the deed. Square in his face.

I was watching. I was not *in* this scene. I'm sure I am now a therapist, and a family therapist at that, partly because the drama in my family resided in this trio that I observed: my mother, my father, and my sister. I looked at all three faces. My father's, covered with pie, was shocked and worried. He was turning toward my mother as if to say, "I never thought she would think I really wanted her to do this to you." My sister's face was wonderfully mobile, traveling between defiance and despair, archness and tears. My mother looked as if she had gotten the pie in her face. She spoke first. In that elegant, calm way she had, correct and in control, she said with conviction, "I will not bake a pie in this house ever again." She turned on her heel, walked into her bedroom, and closed the door.

As I think I understand now, my mother had left my sister with my father, once again, rather than fight to be part of their closeness. My father was still trying to make up for his years away by being playful with Jan, but at the expense of being supportive to his wife's first baking effort. The aggression in my father's and sister's exchange literally drenched the air, but was entirely unacknowledged. My sister acted out her confusion about how to join with her two parents simultaneously.

At the time, I didn't understand any of this. I watched, and reacted emotionally. To this day, I believe that the reach of my father's years away, mediated by ideas people had about the meanings and effects of father absence, shaped our family's life long after he had returned.

Research Perspectives on Father Absence

Although the mental-health community has taken it as axiomatic that father absence is detrimental to the growth and development of children, especially of boys, research studies have rarely focused on this condition directly. One representation of this fact is that much research on fathers in normal child development comes from mothers' reports of paternal behavior, not from fathers themselves.

Recent investigators have tried to understand and go beyond the biases that pervade the literature on fathers. After critically reviewing this literature, Phyllis Bronstein and Carolyn Pape Cowan summarize their conclusions by saying that the fathers' influence has been minimized or ignored when fathers are present in the home, and exaggerated or distorted when fathers are absent. Prior to the 1970s, researchers routinely found the impact of father presence to be minor while finding father absence detrimental.

Newer studies show that fathers contribute to child development in ways that are similar to those of mothers. The findings concerning the impact of father absence are more variable. In some studies, father absence is not strongly associated with negative outcomes, and in others single mothers are described as having particular difficulty handling adolescents, especially sons. Here again, however, these studies may be assuming that physical father absence means no psychological father presence. But this indirect presence seems likely, since the mothers in this study are divorced mothers—that is, mothers in families in which the lingering impact of the father may be great.

The difficulty in specifying the effects of father absence is particularly striking in the literature on divorce. Many researchers have agreed that the negative effects on children of their parents' breakup probably come from several sources, including growing up in a dysfunctional family in the first place, witnessing severe marital conflict over time, and the difficult transition that occurs after divorce. In practice, though, most studies have focused solely on this last source of difficulty. One study, however, looked at a large sample of British and American intact families, and over time studied those families in which divorce occurred. They concluded that the effect of divorce could be predicted by conditions that existed prior to the divorce, when both fathers and mothers were still present.

Obviously, across the many cultures that make up American society, the belief that father absence is a problem is strong. This idea then influences single mothers, who consequently worry that their children, their sons in particular, suffer from the lack of a father. Hoping to compensate the son for his "deprivation" of a father, mothers may become more permissive. Setting insufficient limits may in turn produce challenging behavior in their sons, leading to angry, behavioral escalations. Sons, too, may believe that not having a father in the home is supposed to be a problem. This idea will then intersect with the particular ways not having their father present in the home is a hardship for them. Researchers may be observing the effects of these cultural beliefs about absent fathers as much as the effects of father absence itself.

The Politics of Father Absence: What Does It Obscure?

The contemporary rhetoric of family values, which is a shorthand way of commenting on the importance of fathers and the problems of single mothers, creates another version of the good mother/bad mother split. In this instance, married mothers are good; single ones are bad. There are serious consequences to setting up this split. The rhetoric draws attention away from issues that are at least as pressing as family structure: the violence of adult men toward adult women, for instance; the insufficient supply of jobs that pay enough to support families; homophobia; and the importance of other caregivers to families.

VIOLENCE

American homes are not as safe as America's streets. That is the disturbing conclusion reached by investigators from the Family Violence Research Program at the University of New Hampshire. Working with data from the 1985 National Family Violence Resurvey, they found that almost one in eight husbands carried out one or more acts of violence during the year of the study. Male partners' assaults are 21% more frequent than females', and 42% greater for "severe assaults." That is, a woman may assault her partner once, whereas he is more likely to assault her multiple times. Moreover, the meaning of wife-to-husband assault may be very different from the meaning of husband-to-wife assault. Though the data are insufficiently sensitive to identify the contexts of violence, many researchers speculate that wives' acts of violence are most often self-defense and retaliatory acts. This interpretation is supported by the extremely low rate of assault by women, as compared to men, outside the family.

When women leave families, they are often choosing to leave abusive relationships, or they are choosing to remove children from exposure to violence in their homes. Mothers observe firsthand what researchers are now beginning to document: exposure to marital violence may be the single strongest predictor of, for girls, later vulnerability to violence, and, for boys, later commission of violent acts.

Several years ago I worked with a mother whose adolescent daughter had been caught stealing a car. Both parents were professionals, and none of the four children had ever before committed an antisocial act. The court system treated the theft as an aberrancy, as if it signified nothing. In retrospect the mother felt extremely grateful to her daughter, though at the time, she had felt angry and humiliated by her lawlessness. Later she came to see her daughter's stealing as an act of self-sacrifice. At some level, the daughter felt she had to shake her mother out of her passivity. The mother was a battered wife.

I met with the daughter and her mother; the father refused to attend our sessions. During the first meeting the connection between the car theft and the daughter's rage at both her parents was stunningly clear. By the end of the session the child was in tears and begging the mother to leave her abusive husband. As if she had never considered that she might, the mother later said that in that meeting it was as if she were moving from slow motion to real time. She suddenly understood that it was thinkable and doable to leave.

Some women, having grown up in violent homes, are fearful of living with a man at all. They choose to mother alone rather

than to risk violence. Having seen and experienced maltreatment, they feel better able to protect their children from it
if they parent alone.

Years ago, I visited such a mother in East Harlem. She was
the mother of one of the African-American four-year-olds in my
Head Start class. Lenwood and his mother and three younger
siblings lived in three cramped rooms in public housing, ten
blocks from the program. Lenwood was a slow child and a dear
one. He used to follow me around and look up at me with im-
ploring eyes, hoping I would spend just a little more time with
him than with anyone else. I was crazy about all of the children
that summer, but I did favor Lenwood a little bit: We had a
"relationship."

The day I visited Lenwood's apartment, he was very excited.
His mom had told him I would be coming. To my eye, his home
was both spotless and jumbled. The few objects they had were
stacked on top of each other, accommodating to the facts of little
space and small children.

That Lenwood's mother was pleased to see me is a testament
to how much she attended to her son. A busy woman, overwhelmed, it seemed to me, by routines of child care and survival,
she nonetheless greeted me warmly and interacted pleasantly
throughout the length of my brief visit. She showed an interest
in me, though Lenwood had known me only a short while and
I would be leaving the program soon. When I did leave at the
end of the summer, Lenwood shyly pushed an orange wooden
truck, an inch by half an inch, into my palm. Kneeling down,
looking at a significant part of his worldly possessions, I told
him I would keep it with me always, and I have.

Lenwood's orange truck sits on my desk. It reminds me of
what children need more than anything else; it reminds me that
a youngster who is loved and not maltreated will love. It reminds
me that poverty is not associated with insecure attachment; violence is. Lenwood was what psychologists call a securely
attached child. Securely attached children tend not to get victimized. By age four, Lenwood's mother had given him two precious

gifts: she had loved him and kept him from mistreatment, by her or by others. Though he was vulnerable to the violence all around him, he was safe at home. Having been loved, he could love others; having been given to, he could give to others.

Some single mothers have made this choice for themselves and their children. It is not their single-parent status we should deplore, but the conditions of violence that pertain between men and women and between the haves and the have-nots that form the backdrop for their choice to parent alone.

POVERTY

The current family-values rhetoric focuses on the importance of two parents to support their children economically. This argument is particularly galling to African-Americans who know from experience that marriage is often insufficient to raise a family's income above the poverty line. Though most African-American men and women marry at some point in their lives, marriage does not necessarily solve their financial problems. According to sociologist Christopher Jencks, "the basic reason why blacks are poorer than whites is not that they organize their families the wrong way but that individual blacks earn less money."

Jencks goes on to explain. Despite the assumption of many people that African-American poverty is related to African-American family arrangements, even if all African-American women who headed households were to marry the richest African-American men available, their families would still be "poorer than most." Also, since many unmarried African-American men live with their mothers or sisters, had these men married, their wives might be better off, but their kin might suffer.

Although families with children are more than six times as likely to be poor if headed by a mother alone, marriage will not solve this economic problem. Jobs may. So may helping parents who work at low-wage jobs. Deploring single motherhood takes needed attention away from the very serious problems of unemployment and low income from which far too many families in this country suffer.

HOMOPHOBIA

We have entered an era in which two incomes are usually necessary to support families. Yet there are a variety of ways of establishing a two-income family besides a heterosexual union. What is objectionable to some about these new family forms is that many of them exclude men. That is, they reject the fundamental premise of the absent-father rhetoric: Children suffer without a dad.

Prior to the 1970s, lesbian couples often accepted that premise too. Ideas about the importance of fathers joined ideas about maternal selfishness—in this context, selfishness in depriving a child of a father—to produce an ideological context that has been called the myth of "compulsory childlessness." Lesbians are no longer letting themselves be forced by mainstream culture to give up children because they love women.

Like anyone else, lesbians grow up in the dominant heterosexual culture. It is within this culture that they develop ideas about themselves as lesbian. At many junctures these ideas produce contradictions. For instance, most lesbians were girls before they were aware lesbians, and thus they are subjected to the same pressures of "compulsory motherhood" as girls who choose heterosexuality. For lesbians, the two identities—girl, lesbian— cause strain in contemplating motherhood. Apart from the practical matter of achieving a pregnancy or adopting as a single mother, both very real obstacles not too long ago, there are internal struggles.

All girls learn about the relative value the culture places on being selfless and being selfish. In an era in which popular wisdom expressed the view that lesbian mothers were harmful to children, the very act of contemplating being a mother placed the lesbian in a bind. As Laura Benkov points out in her book on lesbian and gay parents, mainstream culture believes that lesbian mothers assert their selfishness because their children will be the object of homophobic discrimination and will therefore be damaged. The lesbian mother is seen as ultimately responsible for the consequences (presumed to be detrimental) of society's flaws.

The bind is obvious. At the very moment a lesbian believes she is expressing her socially sanctioned desire to mother—women, after all, are supposed to want to mother—she is simultaneously "told" she is wrong. There is a negative injunction in the heart of her positive affirmation. Nor are lesbian mothers subject to disapproval only at the point of choosing to have children. For those women who become or let themselves know about their lesbianism after they have conceived children in heterosexual arrangements, the cultural stigma against lesbianism, as manifested in courts and mental-health institutions, is just as great. Benkov cites the figure that, between 1968 and 1978, 98% of lesbian mothers who were sued for custody lost. Judges assume that it will harm children to see their mother with another woman. Curiously, neither the courts, nor the fathers, seem to imagine that this other woman may become an "other mother" as well. Women who love each other are most likely entering into relationships in which both partners care for the children.

In a culture as relentlessly homophobic as ours, in a culture that privileges women's relationships with males over those with females, mothers who choose to mother with women pay too high a price. This price is based on ideas about absent fathers that may be unfounded. The absent-father rhetoric assumes that when women are not living with men there are no possible fathers for their children—men who can participate with children as role models and companions. By failing to recognize that there can be a strong male presence who is not living in the house, this position denies the important roles played by other men in children's lives—uncles, grandfathers, friends, biological fathers, honorary fathers. By linking itself with homophobic beliefs, the absent-father rhetoric supports the oppression of lesbian women and denies the reality of the other mother for lesbian and other families.

"OTHER MOTHERS"

Focus on an absent father promotes a traditional family form at the expense of considering the strengths of particular families, case by case. If we look at empirical research as well as clinical studies, support for other family groupings besides the mother-father-child family can be found. It is important to remember that, however obscured by the attention paid to absent fathers, if fathers are absent, there can be other adult support for a family: There are "other mothers," who are often, but not always, women.

Harriette McAdoo, a research psychologist, studied 318 African-American single mothers who had full custody of their children. All were employed; half of them had been previously married and half had never been married. They were in their mid-thirties and had an average of two children each.

The single mothers who lived alone had significantly higher levels of stress than those who lived in extended-family environments. On a wide range of measures, there were few significant differences between the groups according to previous marital status. The differences that were found favored the never-married mothers. They had attained significantly higher levels of education and occupational status, and therefore higher incomes.

McAdoo accounts for her findings in a number of ways. First, mothers who never married never lost contact with their extended families. Mothers who had been married were often more isolated, and were therefore forced to interrupt their schooling or employment. Second, never-married mothers did not have to face "the trauma of unhappy marital relationships and the dissolution of marriages." McAdoo concludes that marital status at the birth of a child may be less important than the networks of family support available to a mother at the time of transition to parenthood.

African-American families are not the only ones who have an extended-family tradition, though their tradition is rich and one from which others can profitably learn. I also grew up with a supportive extended family and my sister's and my children did too. I have always had "other mothers" who were caregivers, and my children have also. Yet the language many of us use to acknowledge these relationships is often inadequate, no more so than in the legal domain. Language is connected to social status, which is codified in our laws and legal requirements. Custody is the way we confer status on children's caretakers, and parents are assumed to have custody of children, regardless of whether or not they care for them, unless parents divorce and a legal proceeding specifically removes custodial status. The legal status of a relationship, a status that privileges the two-parent family above any other, may bear little resemblance to the actual caretaking circumstances of a family.

In Perri Klass's novel *Other Women's Children,* she writes heartbreakingly of a grandmother, an other mother, attentively loving and caring for her three-year-old grandson, whose mother has died of AIDS and who is painfully dying himself of the disease. Though the hospital staff largely appreciates Mrs. Wilson's role as Darren's other mother, since she does not have legal custody of the child, she cannot authorize the staff to place a DNR (do not resuscitate) order in his chart. In an infuriating scene, Klass dramatizes the issue for other mothers of having no recognized status in the life of someone they love.

When Darren is dying, the hospital procedure requires that a judge, not his grandmother, make the decision about whether or not life supports can be withdrawn. The judge is not unkind to the grandmother, but he must hear from the assembled doctors, lawyers, and the *guardian ad litem* their views on the best interests of the child. The *guardian ad litem* upholds the claim of the absent father, articulating a current position that the best interests of the child reside with the biological parents, regardless of whether or not the parent has cared for the child. The rights of the absent father become linked to ideas about the importance of fathers per se. In this instance, the meaning and significance of fatherhood become reduced to the fact of a biological connection. The focus on the absent father marginalizes the other mother and threatens, unsuccessfully in the novel, to make biology replace care as the criterion by which we judge adequacy.

The Importance of Fathers

The *guardian ad litem*'s appeal on behalf of the absent father, whose contribution has been his genetic material, dramatizes the hollowness of the political rhetoric of the absent father. The mere existence of the father is extolled by this position, whereas consideration of what his actual presence contributes is ignored. Unfortunately, our *cultural* inattention to fathers, our willingness to treat fathers as inessential to children except as token presences, has had grim and sometimes devastating effects on children, their mothers, and their fathers.

The current Men's Movement, for all its problems—some of which I will discuss—is at least recognizing a serious omission in our cultural consciousness. The Men's Movement has made a compelling case for the importance of fathers to children, particularly sons. Although I find the rhetoric of the movement disturbing and often disagree with the conceptual formulations, nonetheless I value the movement's intention to engage fathers in substantive ways.

In *Iron John: A Book about Men,* Robert Bly states the case that there is "not enough father" for men today. (I will refer to Bly's widely read book as representative of the arguments of the Men's Movement, although it does not address all aspects of this phenomenon.) Bly asserts that men who have not had time to "tune" themselves to masculine frequencies with their fathers will "have father-hunger all their lives." The problem with Bly's presentation of the very reasonable assertion that sons need meaningful relationships with their fathers (and, I would add, fathers need meaningful relationships with their sons) is that he cannot seem to make this case without excluding, diminishing, or demeaning mothers. Though this may not have been his conscious intent, his language and imagery is replete with maternal rejection and hostility.

It seems as though, once again, it is not possible to take a both/and position, to assert that fathers are important without devaluing mothers. And there is an odd disjunction in the Iron John tale: fathers emerge as critical figures at conception and at adolescence, but they are not described as significant during childhood. No, in the Iron John world, "a mother's job is, after all, to civilize the boy." Men are needed to help young men find and keep their hardness; females can only teach softness. It would seem that Bly would like us to believe that if fathers are going to attune their sons to the masculine frequencies they need, certain kinds of activities, like childcare, are out.

In the Iron John world and the public-policy world, childcare is feminine. Embedded in the belief that childcare work is feminine work is the idea that women are available at home to do the childcare. Whereas this may once have been the case for many families, it is no longer so. In 1986, 54% of mothers with children under six were in the labor force, and by the end of the 1990s 75% of women with school-age children will be in the labor force. If fathers are important, which indeed they are, they need to be included in the decision-making about and the provision of childcare.

Currently, the unequal sharing of responsibility for family management has been noted as the single most important cause of marital conflict. Though estimates of time spent with children vary, a recent study reported that fathers spend on average twenty-six minutes per day with children under age six and, as children get older, this investment decreases to an average of sixteen minutes per day. In reviewing research findings on mothers' and fathers' involvement with childcare and household work, the psychologist Faye J. Crosby concludes that men are doing far less than women. In her book *Juggling: The Unexpected Advantages of Balancing Career and Home for Women and Their Families,* she writes: "Compared with women in the post-World War II era, contemporary women appear to have made progress. Compared with contemporary women in some other countries, furthermore, American women appear to be doing well. But in view of the contemporary rhetoric of gender symmetry, rhetoric that men themselves are spouting, the picture seems oddly imbalanced."

The relative lack of involvement of fathers in childcare reflects a serious misunderstanding, in my view, of the importance of fathers. I, too, think that fathers are important and I believe along with Bly that fathers can teach what it means to be masculine to their sons, though I would include daughters as well. We differ in that I believe that masculinity and nurturance are compatible. In fact, I think that the equation of nurturance with softness shows a fundamental misunderstanding of what caring for children entails, and that the separation of masculinity from softness is dangerous.

Take Back Our Homes

Years ago, I joined other women in a demonstration, the slogan for which was "Take Back the Night." The phrase was meant to capture the fear that many women have in public spaces after dark. In writing this book, I have found myself saying, "We must take back our homes." By this I mean that our homes must become places where we feel safe, by day and by night.

I cannot bear that "home" has come to mean to so many the place where your family has privileged access to harm you emotionally, spiritually, physically, and sexually. More than anything else, I would want home to mean the place where people see you, recognize you, listen to you, know you, support you, and love you. The family values that I think are essential are the ones that allow people to feel "at home." It is not the configuration of any family with which I think we should concern ourselves, but the competency of the people there, particularly the adults, to make others, particularly children, feel at home. In this sense then, home is not a place, but a feeling; home can be anywhere, anytime, with anyone.

These days, gay men have been particularly challenged to provide the feeling of home for those they love who are dying of AIDS. Paul Monette, a writer, was a loving partner, companion, "twin," and other mother to his friend Roger Horwitz, who died nineteen months and ten days after his diagnosis of AIDS. In those months and days, Monette cared unstintingly for Horwitz, making him feel at home even in his hospital bed. It is this care that Monette chronicles in *Borrowed Time: An AIDS Memoir*. Walking into his son's room in the hospital after he has died, Roger's father thanks the doctor and, while gripping Paul's shoulder, says, "This boy took care of him like a mother."

It is the father's highest praise, and it is deeply ironic that in commenting on the attentive loving care his son received from a man, he doesn't use himself as the standard; he doesn't say, "This boy took care of him like a father." During my cancer treatment, Hilary also tended me through circumstances that were often grim and filled with bodily fluids I would have preferred to keep to myself. Though it is true that any mother would have been proud to tend her child the way Hilary took care of me, I hardly think that I would honor his devotion by labeling his care "mothering."

We must not only expect fathers to care for children and others, but also recognize their doing so. I would rather the public conversation about absent fathers became one about competent, caring fathers. I would hope that we could all be committed to the kinds of work it would take for this to happen.

Several summers ago, Miranda and I took a long car ride together to visit Ben while he was working as a counselor-in-training at a summer camp. At the beginning of the trip, Miranda put on a cassette tape of the musical score from the show based on *Les Misérables*. She knew that a child's mother dies in the show and for this reason she had been uncertain, at first, whether she would bring the tape for the ride. It was about a year after I had finished treatment. About an hour into the trip, she selected the tape, and, as she had suspected, she began to cry when the child's mother sings the song in which she begs the hero to care for her daughter after she dies. Taking the tape out of the player, tears rolling down her cheeks, Miranda turned to me and said, "Does he do it? Does he take care of her the way she needs? Does she feel loved?"

Thinking about *her* father, I told her the truth. "Yes. He loves her very much. And she feels very loved by him. He takes very good care of her."

"Good," she said. "I feel better."

I think to myself, This must be so. Daughters and sons must
be able to believe that their fathers can love them the way they
need. Daughters and sons must have more than one mother—
other mothers, men and women mothers.

Then I remember the lyrics of a song that the "father" in *Les
Misérables* sings toward the end of the show. He is carrying a
wounded student away from the barricades and he sings a song
whose strongest line is "Bring him home." Home. That word
again.

"Home" has been an important word to me before. When I
got sick, I was very clear about what I needed. Among other
things, I needed my father to be a father in the inclusive way
that I have been speaking about here. I needed my father to tap
into his most nurturing stories about himself and make those
available to me.

We set the tone with each other in the first hour of the visit
he made to me three days after my diagnosis. That visit paral-
leled another visit we had had. When Miranda was born, the
doctors told us she might not live. I was very sick and upset
after her delivery, and Hilary and I asked my father to wait to
see us until after I had more fully recovered from the surgery.
I'm sure the wait was agonizing for him. When he finally arrived,
he sat down on a chair facing me and Miranda, his grandchild,
looked at us, kissed us, and promptly fell asleep for a few moments. During those moments, I was profoundly moved. I understood that he had not slept in three nights and that it was
only in our presence that he could relax enough to fall into
sleep.

I don't think we ever talked together about those moments,
but I have treasured them always. They were moments of intimate connection between us, as I realized the extent to which
he was involved in my worry and hopes for this new child of
ours, and I realized that his caring was as complete in his way
as Hilary's and mine was in our way.

Three years ago, when my father came to see me, we talked
for a while, and then I fell fast asleep on his shoulder, for a few
minutes. I hadn't slept in three nights; so complete was my

worry and fear that nothing could turn it off. When I awoke, we began talking and being together in a way that set the tone for the next year.

Deborah Tannen, in her book *You Just Don't Understand: Women and Men in Conversation,* suggests that men and women speak different dialects, which she calls "genderlects." That is, due to social conditioning, the two genders speak, essentially, a different language. My father and I often have. Tannen says that women speak to make connections and that men speak to assert independence. Women share problems; men solve them. It is a provocative thesis.

Since I am always more interested in the contexts within which behavior happens than the generalities about behavior that can be made, I think that Tannen's thesis is faulty for its lack of specificity of context. In the context of my cancer diagnosis, I shared my "problem" with my father and he listened. Like a woman? Perhaps it is statistically more likely that a woman would listen that way, but why? I think he listened like a woman because he knew he had no solutions to offer. Simple. What could he say to me? What could he solve?

For reasons that I believe I do understand, that day, on my couch, my father shared a description of the problem that was very similar to mine, and both of us were clear that we didn't have the resources to figure it out. Yet. My father offered me the resources at his disposal: his attentive love, his support, and his abundant comfort.

He sustained this relation to me throughout my treatment. He was there when I called at odd hours, there to listen and to take in what I said without offering advice or solutions, and there to share my pain and worry. I am quite sure that his wife was very helpful in supporting his doing this for me, and I am grateful to both of them: to her, for expecting that he could and should, and to him, for wanting and being able to "father" me.

One night, a few weeks after my diagnosis, I had a terrible dream. I am in Cambridge, about twenty years old, and I have just left work to get my car from a parking lot. When I arrive, my car is missing. I look around, and although I see other people whose cars are missing, their loss does not help me with mine. I reflect upon my life, and I realize there is a lot about my life that isn't right. I realize that I have forgotten to study for two subjects and that I'm surely going to fail. This fills me with incredible sorrow. Other people had had such high hopes for me; they had thought I would do a good job, and now I know I will fail, disappointing others and myself. I go to a phone booth and I make a call. My father answers the phone. "Has my report card come?" I ask tremulously. With a voice full of love, he replies softly but clearly, "Just come home."

Home. That is what a father who can "father" can provide a child. This is what a mother can expect a father to provide his child. Fathering is not mothering, though it can be. But fathers and mothers may expect of themselves, and their partners and children may expect of them, that in whatever way a sense of home is conveyed both parents can be responsible for their part of providing this experience.

Home. It is crucial to me that I have a home in which I feel that I am at home, and that I make it a place in which others feel at home too. Yet I feel at home away from my house, with people besides my family. I have felt at home transiently, with people I have barely known. And I have encouraged people I know—clients, friends, my children—to value the moments when they, too, feel at home with people outside their family. In thinking about this position, it is clear to me that I have ideas about what makes a relationship one in which a feeling of being at home can be created. In fact, I may have thought more about the kind of relationship that makes a person feel at home than about anything else in my life. In the last few years, I have articulated my ideas about this, naming this essential quality "intimacy." However, my ideas about intimacy challenge prevailing concepts of intimacy, and it is to a discussion of these concepts that I now turn.

EIGHT

Intimacy with Children

Dismantling Hobbling Ideas about Intimacy

Fourteen was probably Ben's most difficult year for us. It was easy to imagine his story about himself—teenager, hip, old-enough—and hard to put up with it. I missed my cooperative, easygoing son and tangled with my short-fused, provocative one. At the same time, the former Ben was sometimes there and a new, more mature Ben occasionally made an appearance. The metaphor of story, rather than the idea of self, was a great boon to me during this period. I chose to think that Ben was working on his story about himself and that he was undergoing a continual self-editing process. I decided that some days I preferred the changes more than others, but eventually I would like the working draft.

In the meantime, Hilary and I became even clearer about those limits within which Ben's self-story could develop. We were strict about curfews and studying; strict about ways he could get angry; and strict about money. For Ben's part, he argued and stayed within the limits. At fourteen he also decided that he wanted to be a stand-up comic, and I will be forever grateful to him that that difficult year was leavened with some of the funniest times I've ever had.

During the children's winter break that year, we went down to Florida to visit my father and his wife. To my horror, one leg of the trip was on a small commuter flight, and I seriously considered renting a car and driving. Common sense prevailed over panic, and I got on the plane and sat next to Ben. I did fine until just before landing, when I could feel my anxiety shifting to the telltale hypervigilance that signals I am close to panic. Hilary was across the aisle from me. Ordinarily I would turn to him and ask for reassurance, but ordinarily he is sitting next to me.

Instead, I was sitting next to my big son, nearly as tall, weighing at least the same as I. We hadn't had a stellar conversation during the flight—we were both engrossed in our reading—but we had been cordial. What would it signify to him, I thought, if I declined to ask him to comfort me? What story of his would I fit into if I slighted him in favor of his father? What would it say to me about a mother's relationship to her adolescent son?

On impulse, I decided to treat Ben no differently than I would treat a friend. I wanted comfort and I wanted to believe that Ben could and would want to comfort me. I knew that the level of fear I was experiencing was nearly manageable; I could afford to risk asking Ben, not Hilary, for help, and could handle it if Ben was unwilling to deal with me. I wanted to believe that in our ongoing loving relationship, I could ask something of my son that would reveal me intimately to him, even though our relationship hadn't felt particularly close in recent weeks and months.

I turned to Ben. "I'm scared. Could you help me?"

At first he looked puzzled. "How?" he said. "What should I do?"

I took a deep breath and said, "Think about all the times that Daddy and I have comforted you, especially when you were a little boy. You've got tons of memories there, somewhere."

"Oh," he said. He picked up my hand and laid it on my knee. He then began stroking it with his thumb, gently and continuously for the five minutes until we landed.

"Thank you," I said. "That made all the difference."

This exchange had made a difference on many levels. To-gether we made a possibility actual. We proved—albeit just to ourselves—that an adolescent son can comfort and be intimate with his mother in a way that is respectful of each. It was a moment in which the hierarchy of mother takes care of son was temporarily softened as he took care of me. It was a glimpse of all that we had been to each other and all that we could become. I cherish it still.

The episode was truly stirring to me. I realized how close I had come to missing that moment with Ben; how nearly I had chosen to act the way I thought I should and not how I knew I could. The moment crystallized for me the fact that I carried contradictory ideas about the nature of intimacy. There were the ideas that my lived experience provided and there were the ideas I had received from both popular culture and psychological for-mulations. Both were interfering with my relationship to Ben and Miranda. I had to make these received ideas about intimacy explicit to myself, so that I could clarify my own thinking.

It took a while, but my inquiry was eventually productive. I realized I had picked up two distinct ideas about intimacy: in the first, intimacy was a capacity and one could have more or less of it; in the second, people achieved relationships over time that were more or less intimate. Neither idea quite fit how I was living my life, yet these ideas were muddling my thinking. Working backward from my actions, I found that I thought of intimacy as moments of connection, moments when I felt that I had shared something that was important to me while the other person listened and understood me. Or, reciprocally, intimacy developed when someone shared something with me and I lis-tened well and respectfully to that person. For me, intimacy was about sharing feelings, thoughts, wishes, and activities. Rather than thinking of intimacy as desirable but difficult to accom-plish, I realized that I had a kind of rock-bottom faith that it was achievable—with the right kind of effort.

Pushing myself to clarify my thinking about intimacy couldn't have come at a better time, for many forces were arrayed—poised even—to convince me that the intimacy my children and

I had shared when they were young was going to have to stop. They were, after all, moving into and through adolescence. The ideas I had about intimacy intersected with ideas I had about mothering such that, unless I established my approach to this stage, a collision was in the offing.

The intersection came vividly with Ben, since he was my first child to reach puberty. On the plane ride, I worried that asking him to help me might undermine my authority with him just at the time in our life together when he—we—seemed to need it most. I didn't want sharing my vulnerabilities with Ben to affect negatively my ability to invoke a parent-child hierarchy when necessary or, conversely, to undermine his ability to see me as a parent to be reckoned with at times. I needed an idea about relationships that would allow me to move flexibly as the situation warranted, not an idea that described relationships as one sort or another, intimate or not.

Similarly, the idea that intimacy was a capacity wasn't helpful at all. Had I fully accepted that notion, I would never have thought to help Ben find within himself the resources to comfort me. I would have given up the request when he said, "What should I do?"; I would have believed that his question indicated a deficient capacity. Instead, I needed a way to think about the developmental course of his interest in connecting intimately with me. I needed to remember all the glorious moments of his childhood, reminding myself that a child couldn't lose a capacity he once had, though he might choose not to exercise it with his mother.

Inextricably related to the idea that intimacy is a capacity is the belief that boys have less of it than girls. Had I swallowed that notion, I could easily have been discouraged from insisting that Ben could deal with my feelings. If this piece of conventional wisdom, found in psychological formulations as well as popular writing, were true, then I would be expending energy fruitlessly in trying to stay intimate with Ben. Yet I was, and wanted to stay, connected to him.

The Gender Story

Where is it written that boys are less capable of intimacy than girls? It is written in many places, and I call this a gender story. According to this story, boys are considered less able to develop intimate relationships than are girls; mothers are discouraged from sustaining intimate relationships with sons past puberty; and mother-daughter intimacy is touted as having the "materials for the deepest mutuality and the most painful estrangement."

This gender story shows up in many ways. For instance, in the last decade I have heard mothers express disappointment after learning through amniocentesis or ultrasound that they are carrying male fetuses. "I'm afraid I'll never have the closeness with a son that I would have with a daughter," one young woman lamented to me. A more seasoned mother tells me that her fifteen-year-old son is reluctant to go with her to the concert he wants to hear for fear that he will be judged a "mama's boy." A grown-up daughter weeps in therapy, not only because her relationship with her mother is not intimate, but because she feels deprived of what "other daughters have with their mothers. It makes me so jealous when I hear women talk about their mothers with affection. I feel like I'm the only daughter who didn't get my due."

I don't know how recent, or ancient, these gendered ideas about the capacity for intimacy are, but I do know that certain psychoanalytic perspectives have made this point of view explicit. Nancy Chodorow, a psychoanalytically oriented sociologist, may be the most frequently cited exponent of this theoretical view of the gendered capacity for intimacy. I first read her work on this subject before I became pregnant. It greatly influenced my thinking. In her widely acclaimed book *The Reproduction of Mothering,* she attempts to account for the way modern capitalist society creates and re-creates feminine and masculine personalities such that women will be suited to mother and men will be suited to work in the alienating structures of capitalism. Using object-relations theory and Marxism

as her primary theories, she identifies the near universality of
female responsibility for childcare—rather than biological, cultural, or economic factors—as the reason for consistent gendered personality differences.

Focusing on the first three years of life, Chodorow states that
growing girls come to define themselves as like their mothers,
whom they observe relating intimately with them. Boys, on the
other hand, come to define themselves as separate and distinct from their mothers, thus making intimate relationships
appear to be something females but not males care about or
nurture. Chodorow and others who have elaborated on her ideas
believe that this early difference predisposes girls to have greater
potential than boys for participating in intimate relationships.

Chodorow also believes that mothers experience their sons as
more different from themselves than daughters, more "other."
She believes that mothers' differential responses to their male
and female children integrally contribute to what turns out to be
a cycle in which mothering exclusively by females reproduces
the capacity to mother—to be intimate—in daughters but not
in sons.

Before Ben was born, I found her arguments persuasive. After,
with my own feelings on which to draw, her speculations contradicted my lived experience.

In my life, my transformation to being a mother happened
with a son. I fused with the infant Ben, feeling his pain, dream-
ing his dreams, awash in his contentments. In conscious awareness, no connection has ever been as complete for me, nor as
prolonged—not even with my daughter. The very quality of relationship that Chodorow describes for mother and daughter, I
place in my history with my son, my firstborn. I have always
identified this state of "fluid boundaries," as Chodorow calls
them, with my becoming a mother. That is, it was in relation to
my own baby that I felt my boundaries become fluid, temporarily, to allow a profound empathic understanding of his experience. Yet I would never say that this state of fluidity with him
was based on my perception that he and I were alike. Rather, it

came from my giving myself over to the adventure of getting to know him as minutely and completely as I could. Every look, every movement, I noted and absorbed, the better to attune myself to him. And, I venture to say, he watched me too. For me, those early days were profoundly intimate.

Nor was our attunement to each other short-lived. I retained a sense of connectedness to Ben for many years, during which, if someone had asked, I would have said this child, my son, is not "other," though I might not have said he was like me. These two dimensions were not linked for me.

I remember with great clarity the first moment I did experience Ben as other. The moment is clear now, and even at the time I recognized its significance. In retrospect, my image is that it felt as if we had expelled ourselves from the Garden of Eden. As I reconstruct this episode, I see that my willingness to understand and empathize with him broke down. Though the event is trivial, the results were profound.

Ben and a male friend of his pushed Miranda into some shrubbery. Their justification for their behavior clearly signified to me that these boys had absorbed the culture's view of their place in our society. They pulled rank on a girl, not by virtue of greater size or strength or age, ways they had done so in the past, but by virtue of gender. They were emboldened by and authorized by a "superior power" of which they were just starting to get wind. They enacted the classic drama of boy dominates girl. I resented Ben for this and I withdrew my willingness to understand his perspective in this instance.

Seven years had passed before I withdrew from him in this way. It took me seven years to realize that despite our being attuned to each other, there were forces acting on him that were not acting on me. He was getting and acting on messages about how to be a boy that were transforming him in ways that I could follow but not experience. The different messages were serving—and perhaps were even intended—to make it harder for us to understand each other, to shift the ease of intimate connection to one another. Perhaps, too, more insidiously, the messages were setting us up to like each other less.

Feeling this, discouraged, I pulled away from him, subtly, I am sure. I doubt that I am the only mother who has done so. I wonder whether a boy's experience of moments like this in his life is connected to *his* story of voice. That is, could the moments when a mother drops her commitment to understand her son, at whatever age this may happen, be a turning point in voice for him? Is this the moment in which the fate of his voice is sealed?

Once I gave up trying to understand our differences in all matters and pulled away from Ben, what happened? At that point, I began to question whether I wanted to understand him, whether I could understand him, whether I had the requisite experience to encompass the totality of Ben's reality. I inserted more than a sliver of distance between him and me. Timely, yes. He was ready and so was I. Time, too, for him to immerse himself in his peer group. But along with the disruption of my effort to understand him at all times came a "pause" in my relating to him. Where once my responses had been automatic, I now hesitated. I took a pause to consider, to wonder whether I would or would not take him on. A pause long enough, even if a fraction of a second, to convey to this male child that in some subtle way I was confused about how I could and would hold him accountable, could and would try to understand him, could and would let him know what I thought.

Even today, in this pause there is a fraction of a second in which I let him go, set him adrift. It is a moment of deep, though brief, disconnection that I create whenever I perceive him asserting dominance. I associate this with masculine prerogative, and I recoil from trying to understand it. I view him and maintain him as foreign.

Ben was seven when this pause happened the first time. What if he had been seven months or seven weeks or even seven minutes old when I pulled away from him, a male child who had a place in the world I would never have? What would my experience have been like then? Or his? Or ours? Or, put differently, how did I resist so long the cultural pressures to think of him as different and therefore unknowable for as long as I did?

I use this experience to challenge the conclusion many people have come to that men are less capable of intimacy than women due to exclusive mothering of boy babies by persons of the opposite gender. I don't feel that my *mothering* of Ben created a different capacity in him for intimate sharing, but, rather, that as he got older he picked up ideas from the culture that began to separate us. I didn't share those same ideas with him, and I didn't like them or want to understand them either. It wasn't our differences per se that interfered with our intimate connection, but my unwillingness and disinterest, his unwillingness and disinterest, in bridging the differences.

Difference doesn't inevitably divide. I know that from loving Hilary. On the contrary, turning what at first seems strange into something familiar is one of the most important opportunities we have in caring for others. It is a process that creates the feeling of intimacy. Had I tried to understand what Ben liked about pushing Miranda into the shrubbery (and had he tried to understand why I felt it abhorrent); had I thought that talking together might lead us both to modify our positions; had I believed that he could be dislodged from behaving aggressively that moment need not have disrupted our intimate connection with one another. But I did not, and it did.

Metaphors of Closeness and Distance

I have also begun to think that a common synonym for intimacy, "closeness," influences mothers' behavior with their sons and daughters. Take the popular ditty "A daughter's a daughter all of her life, a son's a son 'til he takes a wife." On the surface, this seems to be the regretting of a fact from the mother's point of view. I think there is also an embedded injunction here, warning mothers that they must not attempt to keep their sons close to them throughout their lives.

Robert Bly, in *Iron John,* seems to ally himself with the underlying message of this popular saying when he writes that distance between mothers and sons is necessary at puberty. Blaming older men for their failures to "interrupt the mother-son unity" at adolescence, he writes: "A clean break from the mother is crucial."

Why is it fine for girls but not boys to remain intimate with their mothers, and what does the language of closeness conjure up that is disturbing in relation to boys? One objection, I think, is a political one. Boys mustn't remain close to their mothers because mothers are not the people from whom boys can learn how to take their proper place in the social order. Since boys must be able to dominate women, and since mothers are "superior" to sons in the generational hierarchy, closeness to the mother will produce unworkable binds for the mother-son relationship. Distance is the preferred solution. Daughters, on the other hand, can stay close, because their "proper" place is precisely to learn from their mothers how to tend to hearth and home.

A second basis for objection is sexual. Mothers and sons must put distance between each other at puberty to control the sexual attraction between them. Shades of Oedipus and Jocasta. Yet intertwined with concern about potential sexual impropriety may lurk another layer of distress. In a sexual encounter with his mother, an adolescent boy would not be the dominant partner—as a male "should" be in a sexual encounter. This adds a political dimension to the feared sexual violation.

Curiously, mother-daughter closeness doesn't seem to conjure up the same kind of worry in most people. I suspect that the absence of a clear prohibition or even concern reflects a deepseated homophobia based on a denial of sexual desire between women. Clearly, I am not advocating sexual intimacy between mothers and their sons or daughters, but only observing how different the concern over closeness between mothers and sons seems to be from that over mothers and daughters.

I get a terrible sinking feeling when I consider how often and in how many ways I and other mothers receive the message that closeness to our maturing sons is "bad" or "inappropriate." A few weeks ago, I attended a track meet of Ben's, and when he finished his race, he slumped onto my shoulder and we walked together during his cool-down. Before separating, he gave me a hug and then walked away to join his team. Two women I had never met made a point of coming over to tell me how "unusual" my son was to "let" me hug him in public. Though their tone was complimentary, even wistful, perhaps, the subtext was clear: boys don't act that way with mothers.

I have grave concerns that a culture that encourages mothers to pull away from their adolescent sons may be inadvertently contributing to the escalation in male violence we are so desperate to stop. Studies of men who are violent to their female partners consistently report that a primary reason for these acts of aggression is fear of abandonment even if the purpose of the aggression is intimidation. Is it not likely that cultural messages that encourage mothers and sons to distance themselves from each other, as the way to manage intimacy, produce the very feelings of abandonment that men then handle by attempting to dominate the women they erroneously believe they are entitled to control? Men's violence to their female partners is a serious public health problem. I am not making light of this in proposing that targeting prevailing ideas about the mother-son relationship might be an effective prevention strategy, along with the many others that need to be tried. Mothers and sons need a way to feel good about continued, sustained, nonintrusive, nonsexualized intimacy. Mothers and sons need to feel entitled to this in order to work for it.

Several years ago I worked with a sixty-five-year-old woman whose husband had recently sued her for divorce. They had been married for thirty-five years and had four children, three daughters and a son. For most of those years, the marriage had been a good one, but the last several years had been troubled. Although not surprised, the woman was shocked that her husband would take the unilateral action of suing her for divorce without discussing his plan to do so with her. She found herself wanting to scream and rage and throw things. Work soothed her, as did the friendships she had nurtured with men and women over the years.

Her three daughters stayed in regular touch with her and their father. As the Christmas holidays approached, each daughter made plans to visit each parent separately. Her son, however, did not call her, and she learned through one of her daughters that he had said, "I can't handle it," and that he planned to visit a friend's parents during the holidays.

In discussing with the mother her feelings about the children, I asked questions to highlight the differences in the daughters' and the son's behavior and puzzled with her about what could account for this. The mother was perplexed and disturbed by her son's response, since she had felt equally "intimate" with him and her daughters. She explained that she and her son shared a number of interests and that he was the child with whom she still did the most—they went birding together, for instance.

Hurt by her son, she believed there was nothing she could do about it. I asked her to try to articulate why she thought she couldn't do anything about it. In her inner scenario, her son was vulnerable. He was suffering because of the divorce and he needed distance. If she talked to him, he would feel criticized, pushed, and nagged by her. He would feel violated by her, intruded upon.

I then asked her what she thought her daughters felt now? What could she take up with them? Why were her assumptions and expectations with respect to sons and daughters so different? Where, I said, with an attempt at humor, is it written on the "Y" chromosome that daughters, but not sons, support their mothers during a divorce?

I felt that not only were differential expectations based on gender-related ideas at play here, but also the very language of closeness and distance was obscuring distinctions that were important to make. In our conversations I tried to introduce these. For instance, did she want him to be "close" to her, or just be "in touch"? Was it the lack of heart-to-heart conversation that bothered her, or his failure to be in contact at all?

She decided she would call him. We discussed words and tone. I asked her whether she was clear about what she wanted from her son. Was it something that in other circumstances he would be easily able to offer another person, or did she want something that would be a stretch for him in any situation? She clarified for herself that she didn't want to talk with him about her feelings and problems, but, rather, wanted to know that he cared about her, which he could signal by calling periodically to ask after her.

She did talk to her son. She told him that his support would mean a lot to her at this time and that if he could check in with her periodically she would appreciate it. He told her he would try to do that.

She did not let him go; she moved through "the pause." She came to believe that there were ways for her son to take emotional space for himself without hurting her in the process. She dropped the double standard for her son that had surfaced in the aftermath of the great vulnerability she had felt upon being served divorce papers. By distinguishing what felt nonintimate— her son's withdrawing from all contact with her—from his reasonable wish to take time to integrate what his parents' divorce meant to him, they were able to realign their relationship. The metaphor of closeness-distance—the words themselves—had made it harder, not easier, for this mother to think her way through to what she felt entitled to from her son.

Talk about Relationships

I have also noticed, and since noticing I would now say I am keenly aware, that there is a subtle bias about what kinds of topics qualify as ones around which intimacy forms. It has been my observation that *talking about relationships* has become the gold standard for deciding whether or not a conversation—even a relationship—is intimate. This makes the content of a conversation the key to its intimate or nonintimate nature, but in my view what people talk about is less important than whether each person feels included in whatever they are doing together. When talking about relationships is taken as the measure of intimacy, anything else is less good or avoidance.

This contradicts what any mother knows about how intimacy happens with children: talking about relationships is surely not the be-all and end-all of intimacy. Children rarely talk about relationships, and yet mothers commonly feel intimate with them. I think that intimacy with children happens through relating synchronously during any activity, whether blowing bubbles, counting macaroni, going ice-skating, watching a videotape, or chatting in the car.

Yet I do get tripped on occasion, thinking that talking about relationships is the best way to generate intimacy, rather than the way with which I am most at ease. Nor am I alone in this. Research studies have shown that girls and women say they enjoy talking about relationships more than do men. This difference emerges as early as four and a half, at which age boys' and girls' interest patterns and interactive styles begin to diverge. The idea, however, that one set of interests and one style is more likely to produce intimacy seems to me to be part of the problem, not the solution. It also creates a standard that favors females in this culture.

Depending on how the people involved feel about what they are doing together—watching a sporting event, listening to music, going fishing, cooking a meal, reading a story aloud, driving in a car, discussing a problem, building a desk—talking about a relationship can be an intimate or nonintimate experience. Nor is it likely that an observer could tell whether others are sharing intimately with each other. What passing person would have said that the older gentleman slumped in sleep on the molded plastic chair in the new mother's hospital room was providing his daughter with one of her most memorable moments of intimacy?

Feeling intimate with others occurs through learning about and then participating in others' interests and excitements— their passions. Or, as with my father, it comes about through showing that you care as deeply about someone or something as the other person does. I could have missed the fact that he was showing me how much he cared if I had believed that only spoken words can communicate thoughts and feelings.

But intimacy is tricky. Developing intimacy requires a certain amount of negotiation, explicit or not. If one way a woman experiences intimacy is talking about relationships, then any man who wants to be intimate with her may choose to develop an interest in this as well. If a boy is in a particular phase in which he experiences intimacy by laughing with his buddies at the movies, then anyone who wants to be intimate with him may decide to go with him to the movies. If a young girl loves roughhousing and hates reading, then the parent who wants to be intimate with her may, for example, elect to overcome his or her fastidiousness in order to wrestle her. If a man loves sitting in a rowboat fishing, then those who wish to be intimate with him may find themselves in the same boat.

Thus, if a mother wants to be intimate with her children, she may have to do things she wouldn't ordinarily imagine herself doing. I'm not interested in sports, but Ben is. For a time, I got up early and read the sports pages before Ben came down to breakfast. I learned quickly that, although he got a kick out of my growing astuteness about the world of baseball and basketball, morning was not a good time to talk. Though I must say my commitment to staying current with his favorite teams' successes and misadventures has waned over time, I treasure the memory of a heated argument about a Red Sox trade as much as that of a private dinner we had talking about "us."

Intimacy and Stage Theories

Though the gender story, in its many facets, is a critical element influencing many mothers' ideas about intimacy with their children, so, too, I think, is the idea that intimacy is a final *stage* of relationship, reached by only some mature couples who are already capable of consistent mutuality. Though obviously this stage-based idea of intimacy is intended to describe the relationship between adult couples, elements of the idea may seep into mothers' thinking about intimacy with their children, producing confusion.

A stage-based view of intimacy produces conundrums when applied to children. My children and I have certainly not reached a "stage" of consistent mutuality with each other, though we have had years of sweet sharing. We have shared patty-cakes gone haywire, wordless nuzzles at bedtime, and the decoding of Hebrew letters. The idea of intimacy as a late stage of relationship would discredit mother-child intimacy in childhood and provide a rationale for accepting a lack of intimacy during adolescence.

Nor does the idea of intimacy as a stage of relationship help to explain the intermittent quality of intimacy that many mothers experience with their children. Moment to moment the quality of connection may slip from harmony to discord, intimacy to estrangement, understanding to misunderstanding. If intimacy is a stage of relationship, and there has been intimacy at one point, then how can we account for the long periods that many mothers go through with their children when nothing clicks and all seems hopelessly conflictual?

I think the continual changes in children's growth and development account for the uneven rhythms of intimacy that mothers experience with them. These changes, too, are frequently described as stages, and I don't think that the concept of a stage is helpful in this regard either. Stages are fixed, at least for a period of time. Yet even within long stretches of conflict, moments of intimacy can happen. Especially if one has faith that this can be so. Unwittingly, stage theories may make us miss opportunities to create intimacy out of the meager openings children provide.

Thoughts about Intimacy and Its Opposite

As I have been suggesting, I fear that thinking of intimacy either as an individual's capacity that is determined early in life or as a stage of a relationship actually makes it harder to achieve. I think of intimacy as something that people can create with each other at any time, if they are open to sharing what they truly care about and open to trying to understand what the other finds meaningful. This can happen in any relationship—with children, friends, clients, or strangers—but it surely doesn't always occur. In order to grasp what another person means, you have to really *listen* to that person. This, it turns out, is exceedingly difficult to do. We often think we understand someone else when we actually understand the sense *we* have made of what that person has said.

There is a wonderful simple exercise that a legendary family therapist, Virginia Satir, used to illustrate this point. She would ask one person to talk briefly to another about himself. Then the listener was asked to reflect back to the speaker what he had said in the form of a question that began, "Do you mean . . . ?" The listener often had a revelatory experience. Most people assumed that they did know exactly what the other meant and were taken aback if they received a negative response.

As a therapist, I have trained myself to believe that I don't understand what people mean. I have trained myself to no longer think that saying to someone "I know exactly what you mean" is of benefit. I believe, instead, that my job is to create the conditions for us to develop an understanding together of what is meant. The meanings that emerge from the collaboration of therapy offer new possibilities for feeling, thought, and action. Listening this way is a skill. The trick for me has been to use this skill as a parent.

It sometimes happens that in order to understand another person the listener has to commit herself to the arduous process of not understanding too quickly, so that the speaker can discover through her own speaking what she thinks or feels. The speaker needs to believe that her listener is willing to suspend what she thinks she knows in order to hear what the speaker wishes to be so. This is a magical enterprise. Invited, as I am as a therapist, to go through such sacred conversations daily, I feel truly privileged. There is no other work I would rather do. As a parent, I know how effective this way of listening can be, and yet I frequently take a shortcut and act as if I know what my kids mean without letting them tell me themselves.

I don't want to overemphasize the importance of talk. As I have pointed out, intimacy often doesn't involve talk at all. Speaking is just one way people can share what's important to them. Touch, gesture, action, and writing are also ways that people share what's meaningful to them. When my children were little, I felt incredibly "intimate" with them when we would play, for example, mirroring games with each other—both matching and varying our gestures in what felt like the most exquisite connectedness. Even as they get older, intimate moments are often nonverbal.

Once, when Miranda was eleven, she had minor surgery that required general anesthesia. In the aftermath, she had a lot of discomfort, and over the course of several hours my attention faltered. I became impatient and bored. She spent the afternoon moaning and eating red Jello. Her surgeon had insisted that she and I could go to a play that evening. We went despite my misgivings, because Miranda was eager to do so. During intermission, out on the lawn on a lovely summer's evening, she began vomiting. She vomited larger quantities than I have ever seen in my life, which is saying a great deal. Both of us were covered. Just as she started to feel better, but before either of us was clean, and on the periphery of what I can only imagine must have been a horrified group of spectators, we began to laugh so hard that we were holding on to each other to keep from falling over. In this moment, I felt intimate with Miranda, because of the realization that we were both people who could respond to this disgusting situation with humor.

I think that intimacy happens when there are repeated intimate moments that aren't overwhelmed by nonintimate ones, so that over time people feel known to each other. According to this view, for a mother to be intimate with her child she must be willing to let herself be known. For some mothers—mothers like me who grew up believing that we had to be "selfless"; mothers who believe that maintaining a position of authority in every situation is fundamental to good parenting; mothers who fear burdening their children—letting themselves be known, sharing stories of who they really feel themselves to be, is challenging. In fact, it is the heart of the matter of intimacy.

It may be precisely at the times we are most uncomfortable with our own feelings that we pull away from our children, thinking that we are protecting them by concealing ourselves from them. I stopped sharing my feelings and thoughts with my children during the time when we were waiting for the lab results that would influence the next plan of action: mastectomy, chemotherapy, or radiation. Hilary and I would huddle in our bedroom, as often as possible after the children had gone to bed, to ponder likely recommendations and our reactions to them. Often Miranda, then age nine, would get out of bed and require attention for some minor but seemingly contrived complaint. It drove me wild. Knowing this period was as hard for her as for me, I knew I should respond sympathetically. But my heart hardened to her each time she interrupted my time with Hilary—time I desperately needed, to go over and over, obsessively, this outcome or that.

One night, unable to contain myself, unable to let the more patient Hilary deal with her, I exploded at her. "Please, can't you let us alone?" I yelled in a desperate, beseeching tone of voice.

As if struck, she ran to her room, sobbing hysterically, with me, furious and penitent, behind her. After considerable time, Miranda stopped crying, and, while still breathing unevenly, she talked about how isolated she felt. "You want me to tell you everything, but now you won't tell me anything," she charged.

"We've told you," I replied, covering my distress with the measured calmness I affect if I want to appear in control when I am not, "that as soon as we know what is going to happen next, we will tell you."

"That's not what I mean," she insisted, as if I were really dense. "I want to know everything now. I get scared when you don't tell me everything that's going on."

"But nothing *is* going on," I responded obtusely.

"Then why do you and Daddy talk to each other so much and nobody talks to me?"

I was silent. She had captured my attention and at that instant I began to listen to what she was saying very carefully. As can happen, the shift in my attention signaled a different kind of listening on my part, and a space opened up for Miranda to speak to the core of her pain. "I feel like all my life I've been a person who helped other people when they were in trouble and now I feel like *I'm* drowning in a river and people are just prancing by," she said.

Stunned, I looked at her for a long puzzled moment. "People? Do you mean me?"

"Yes," she replied. "You don't talk to me anymore."

"I think I have been talking less to you, but what I have to say, what I say to Daddy, is about feelings that I don't think would be good for you to hear, that I'm not sure I'm comfortable sharing with you."

"But I want to know everything. You're leaving me out and I hate that."

Miranda insisted that she would rather be overwhelmed at times with feelings and ideas beyond her capacity to integrate, in exchange for feeling included. Hilary and I, in our effort to "spare" her, were making her feel less, not more, in control. To respond honestly to her request, I had to say things to her that I thought a mother ought not to. I had to tell her that I was scared. I had to tell her that I was furious at the person who lost my slides and dragged out the tumor analysis by an extra four weeks.

In opening up to Miranda, I had to confront my fears that confiding in her would blur a generational boundary between us that I wanted to keep in place. I learned to accept that when she wanted me to talk to her, we could decide together what extent of conversation worked for us both. Often, early on, I couldn't bear to reveal the extent of my pain to her. I desperately needed privacy. She didn't really need for me to tell her all that I was feeling, but, rather, to know that I was having intense painful feelings. This made her feel less alone. Our collaboration felt mutual, and respectful of my wish that there be only one grownup in the exchange. By not shielding her from parts of myself with which I felt uncomfortable, I let her be more comfortable, as she had predicted. For Miranda, though not for Ben, that was the better choice.

This episode underscored for me that sharing yourself with someone is intimate only when it is mutually desired. The agreement we made with one another allowed me to feel good about myself as a mother and good about the way I was taking care of my own needs, whether I told her I didn't want to talk to her or I did talk to her.

More recently, it seems to me that I am the one who is more likely to want to talk about myself, and she is the one who is not interested. When I am the one who wants to talk about myself and neither Ben nor Miranda seems interested, or when they are actively showing me that they are uncomfortable, then sharing my feelings or my thinking is no longer an intimate act. It's intrusive, off-putting and nonintimate. And I have to admit that, initially, I experienced Miranda as imposing on me when she asked me to disclose my feelings to her during the early days of my cancer treatment. Fortunately, we were able to work it out so that her desire stopped feeling like a demand.

Mutual sharing seems to create intimacy, and imposing one's views or feelings or actions on others seems to create the opposite. Some mothers do tell more to their children more often than their children can bear. Regardless of the intimate nature of the content, this kind of speaking does not produce intimacy.

Nonintimate behavior happens in all kinds of ways, some of which are essential to family life. Parents of children must be able, for example, to impose meaning on their children for their own safety ("You may not cross the street unless you are holding a grown-up's hand") or to tell children what to do ("Always wash the fruit before you put it in the refrigerator") and what not to do ("You may not hit me").

Not all impositions are problematic to the person on whom they are imposed. Hours after my mother died, I returned to my sister's apartment and gratefully roused an already stirring Ben to nurse him. I turned toward Ben feelings that were as much about my mother's loss as about his presence. Coming from the saddest vigil of my life, I imposed on him feelings and meanings far beyond his ken. Watching his breathing, I couldn't help but superimpose the image of my mother's final breaths. I was filled with awe at the human condition, which sometimes arranges the perfect comfort in the deepest pain. Did the tenderness and intensity of expectation I felt lifting his tiny body and pressing him to my heart harm him? I think not.

Not all such impositions are so benign. Telling your child accurate stories of your life's pain when the child has not chosen to be your witness harms children, even as it underscores your need. Telling your child you understand him when you don't is confusing to the child, who may or may not be able to defend his perception that he is misunderstood. When children are repeatedly misunderstood, they come to doubt their own reality. This is serious indeed. Sometimes an activity that starts out as consensual degenerates into one that is unilateral. A mutual cuddle that becomes a sexual assault will have devastating effects. Imposing on another, not taking the other's needs into account while gratifying one's own, can produce much pain, making family life unbearable. Though any family member may be guilty of doing this, there are particular difficulties when parents do, for they are the people children love most and on whom they depend. Parents have the power, and children are rarely able to confront their parents when real harm is being done to them. The dynamics of power and fear, so intermingled in abuse, create deep and devastating silences that can last decades and beyond.

When parental imposition doesn't *massively* disregard the child, children are more apt, sooner or later, to challenge the parental dictum. These challenges are the moments when parents and children alike learn whether the child is ready to enter a more mutual relation with the parent. Both the parent and the child must be worthy. These are the exchanges in which children take their place alongside their parents, allies for the moment in working together for what is in everybody's best interest. These are the moments in which both parent and child have a measure of the child's developing maturity.

Take the rule "You may not go out after dark." I remember when Ben and I moved beyond this rule.

"Mom, that's a stupid rule," he said. "All my friends take the MBTA at night."

"Ben, four of your friends were beaten up waiting for the train at night. I am not going to get into this with you. I am not negotiable here."

These were our opening moves. I was waiting to see what Ben did next. If he backed down—given the fact that our relationship is a continuously changing one with each other—I would infer that he was not really ready to go out at night, that he was just testing the waters. If, on the other hand, he pursued me, I would know that it might be time for us to renegotiate the rule.

He came back. "I don't think you're being fair. I'm only talking about going to the movies and back, and I would go with a friend."

"That's just what those boys were doing when they got beaten up."

"What if I take the train in the opposite direction, so I have to stand on another side of the platform, and then I go to a safer stop and cross over and come home?"

I knew that something was afoot. It was likely that he really did feel ready to take on the risk of riding the train at night. I told him that, although that plan wouldn't work, maybe there was another possibility. What if he had permission to go to one movie house, the one next to the safer train station, and not the other? That was fine with him. We created a new rule, but actually the "ruleness" of it dissolved. Ben and I were on the same wavelength.

Cumulatively, exchanges like this make me feel intimate with him. We work together, mutually, to set forth our needs and to respect the other's needs. This is a process that we have gone through a zillion times already, and I trust that we will continue to go through a zillion times more. In this instance I was aware that certain ways of behaving were likely to make us feel greater understanding of each other and that certain other ways were likely to estrange us. Perhaps even more critical, though, was the fact that no matter where this conversation might take us, I felt confident that there was nothing I would have to reveal to Ben that would make me feel bad about myself, or bad about myself as a mother. The heart of the matter for me was that I was concerned about his safety. I might disclose that I handled this maternal concern with more anxiety than some other mothers, but that wouldn't violate my idea of what was acceptable for a mother to feel. I am more likely to fall out of intimate connection with my children when I fear they will learn something about me that I judge negatively or when I fear they will learn something that I deem them "too young" to know. I must guard against excessive restraint in order to foster intimacy.

So What's a Mother to Do?

This, then, is one of the central dilemmas of voice: to speak not just what is acceptable to oneself and others, but to speak that which is not, or may not be, acceptable. If we don't challenge ourselves to go beyond the limits of what we assume a mother "should" reveal, if we "choose" silence, we will cut ourselves off from the richest intimacies we can have with our children.

The challenge is immense. We must overcome our own inhibitions as well as the constraints that prevailing cultural norms would place on us. At the same time, we must teach our children to tolerate letting us be more authentic by exposing them to our points of view, our experiences, incrementally, in developmentally appropriate ways.

Nor will we always get it right. In trying to be more intimate with our children, nonintimate moments are bound to happen. The inevitable lapses that arise can become opportunities for reestablishing intimate contact. I don't think we can make commitments to understand others, only to *try* to understand them. I think the process of moving toward understanding another is what produces intimacy in the first place, including intimacy between mothers and their sons or daughters.

I believe that mothers should be encouraged to stay in intimate connection with their sons and daughters throughout their lifetimes. However, what I mean by "intimate" relation requires constant, concerted effort to stay in contact in ways that are *mu-*

tually agreeable and satisfying. Intrusion and intimacy are opposites.

There is yet another aspect to this matter of intimacy. Mothers—and would that fathers were too—are strategically placed in families to do essential teaching about what constitutes intimate and nonintimate ways of behaving. I firmly believe that children can be taught to protect themselves from all kinds of abuse if they have been taught to recognize when someone is imposing ideas, feelings, plans, or wishes on them. Many families teach children to respect others, but I would prefer that lesson to come with an add-on: respect others as long as they respect you. When they do not, you need to notice in what ways they are showing disrespect. Are they disrespecting you by imposing on you in ways that make you feel scared or weird or hurt or uncomfortable? Are they imposing on you by asking you to keep a secret from people with whom you normally share your experiences?

Although these may not be the lessons every mother wants to teach her children, I fear that avoiding this kind of education endangers our children. By teaching children that they are entitled to be in relationships that make them feel safe, we will be protecting them while learning crucial lessons ourselves.

A questioning child is not a docile one. I know, because I have two children who challenge. They are adolescents now and issues of separation are entwining themselves into the center of our intimate life together. Age is combining with upbringing and temperament to create a whole new level of give and take, stay and go, back and forth. Understanding separation, so infused and confused with issues of loss for me, is the final piece of work I have set myself to do.

Timely. I see my oncologist tomorrow. Carving up my year into six equal pieces of time, these appointments raise the question of whether I will get to finish that which I want to do. I tell myself that I will deal with separation whether the news this time is good or not, for separation is an issue that no family is able to avoid.

NINE

Growing Up, Not Apart

My Post-Treatment "Adolescence"

Reprieve from my oncologist. No disaster this time. My doctor, for the first time ever, shakes my hand and tells me I have done a good job, as if my hard work could keep the cancer cells at bay. Although he knows that I would do anything to keep the checkups lump-free, there is little I can do. Nor has my post-treatment course been simple or straight. I have had other lumps, other spots, other X rays, other operations. Each exacts its toll.

During the first few months after treatment ended in August 1989, I was weak, broken, and silent. Like a person who has suffered a trauma, I had symptoms of hyperarousal, intrusive thoughts, and numbness. Anxious and hypervigilant, alert to any mentions of cancer, dying, or death, I found daily life a continuous assault. I rarely slept through the night, but would wake from a nightmare, dripping with sweat. The worse I felt, the worse I thought I was. I made blame a vortex and descended into its center, boring lower and lower. In that state, I could imagine no good coming from continuing contact between my children and me. I pulled away.

I pulled away to the extent that the mother who shopped, cooked, drove, did errands, disciplined, and monitored home-

work was present as a shell; the mother who had always ani-
mated these tasks was far away. I could not stay connected,
partly because I felt I should not stay connected. What if I were
to die? What if the next scheduled checkup showed that, without the chemotherapy, cells had begun to proliferate? Or that
cells had merely hidden from the rads and chemicals, and were
now coming out from hiding, ready to grow and gambol again?
If this were so, if this were to be so, I reasoned, if I might die
and leave my children (my husband, my family, my friends, my
colleagues), might it not be better for all of us if I backed away
now, saving them and me the pain of severing rich connections?

I tried this out. I was not loving or lovable—especially and
particularly with the people who seemed to want me the most.
These people, I reasoned—those who showed me how much
they would care were I to die—needed to detach from me the
most. Perhaps, I thought, getting into practice for the eventuality
might help.

That logic expressed ways of thinking and feeling about separation that were truly from another era, before my own clinical
work and theorizing had begun to shift received ideas I had
about what separation is and what one can do about it. In this
vulnerable time, my thinking returned to older ideas, other people's formulations, and I lost the courage of my own.

I take it as a great and good fortune that my children were
entering adolescence—Ben already there, Miranda steps away.
Watching and learning from my relationships to them—both in
relation to their developmental shifts and my own experiences
living with an uncertain future—has brought me back to the
perspective on separation I had developed as an adult and as a
therapist, before I got cancer. It has helped me sharpen the critique of existing ideas about separation that I carried inside me,
ideas that I read, heard, and saw enacted in family and therapeutic relationships all around me.

It is intriguing to me that, in the aftermath of cancer treatment, in the context of a belief that I might have to detach myself from my family and leave them, I developed a style not too
dissimilar from that of many adolescents on the brink of leaving

home. Although I doubt anyone would ever have called me sullen, I was withdrawn, moody, and irritable. And although surely there was a lot more going on than just the fear that I would have to leave—die—the parallel was striking enough for me to try to learn as much as I could from it.

Traditional Ideas about Separation

As a clinician in training, I was taught two principle ways of thinking about separation. Though there are important differences between them, they have in common that they are theories based on infant, not adolescent, observation. Curiously, they have formed the backdrop for much clinical understanding of the separation of adolescents from their families of origin.

One of the theories I learned focused on the effects on infant attachment of early deprivation from primary caretakers. This work emphasized that the infant was not passive but required the involvement of caretakers, particularly the mother, for development to proceed positively. In contrast, the other theory emphasized the infant's individualism. The infant's development was conceptualized as proceeding from symbiotic merger with the mother to individuation, from conjoined oneness to single oneness. Though acknowledging the importance of the mother in caring for the infant, this theory depicted the developmental pathway as a movement away from fusion to a distinct separateness.

The first theory lays the foundations for theorizing about the importance of connectedness for maturity. The second theory lays the foundations for theorizing about the importance of autonomy as the sign of maturity. Theorizing about adolescence reflects these two perspectives. Whereas both perspectives identify developmental tasks associated with adolescence, such as forming an identity, becoming competent in skills that will permit independent living, and forming intimate relationships, they differ in their descriptions of the ideal process by which these tasks are accomplished—the one emphasizing connectedness, the other autonomy.

These two perspectives on adolescence have one major characteristic in common: neither imagines the mother—or father, for that matter—as an active player during this stage. For the most part, parents are not discussed at all, or if they are they figure as backdrop to the more central drama happening on the stage—that is, the adolescent's development. Few theories of adolescence place the child in the context of his or her family, or recognize that the parents are developing too. By omitting the parents from theorizing, our understanding of adolescence is greatly narrowed, for not only, in my view, do parents experience their own continual process of development, but they are influenced by their adolescents' growth as well.

Imagining parents as integrally related to the adolescent's process of development precisely because the parent, too, is continuing to develop recasts the meaning of separation at adolescence. Whereas traditional theories see adolescence as a time of individual identity formation—or individuation—for the young person, I see it as a time of mutual change for parent and child. Where traditional theories stress independence as the primary goal of the period, I see "mutual knowing" as a goal as well. And, there is also the matter of leaving. Yes, adolescents leave, but their leaving, unlike the departures of those who die, can represent gain, not loss, to the entire family. Adolescents go away, but they can return with rich interests and connections to share.

Separation as Mutual Change

ADOLESCENCE

Adolescence has been called the "second individuation phase" to underscore the continuities with the first stage of individuation, at which time the infant is believed to emerge from a symbiotic fusion with the mother. By using this name, theorists emphasize the resonances between the infant's and the adolescent's separation work, implicitly linking the adolescent's development of identity, intimacy, and competencies with a break from parents.

Perhaps no current popular book is as explicit about the break from the parents as Robert Bly's *Iron John*. (Again, I refer to this book because it is representative of a way of thinking, not because it is the only instance of it.) The book champions a boy's break from his mother at adolescence. There are two story lines in *Iron John*—one, mythological; the other, a contemporary application of the myth. In the contemporary story line, as I have said earlier, Bly writes that "a clean break from the mother is crucial." In the mythological tale, the boy steals the key to the Wild Man's cage from under his mother's pillow. Though Bly is at pains to describe why the boy is required to steal the key from his mother, his logic rests on a premise that I challenge. Bly tells us that "the possessiveness that mothers typically exercise on sons . . . can never be underestimated." Mothers, he says, would never give away the key because they are "intuitively aware of what would happen if he got the key: they would lose their boys."

Bly's theorizing is based on at least two assumptions with which I disagree: one has to do with mothers and the other with separation. Bly conceptualizes the mother as static, a person whose own development has stopped and who is dependent on her son for a vital connection to life. This mother fears the boy's changes, for she sees difference as threatening, not exciting. Bly does not imagine a mother with whom I can identify, a mother whose son is part of, but not all of, her life's canvas.

As for separation, Bly's version equates separation with a rupture. He does not imagine a process by which the son's relationship with the mother is ongoing while he experiments, as he must, with activities of his own. In Bly's view of adolescence, separation must be a "clean break," because he cannot imagine a mother who would be interested in and not intrusive about her son's discoveries.

In an Iron John world, I would have to resign myself to becoming an insignificant person in Ben's life. Not only would this violate how I imagine our future together, but it would violate the critical work I have done so far. I became a mother with Ben. I have already figured out that mothering him is part of my journey but certainly not all. I have already figured out how to mother and continue on my path. Now Bly would have me get off Ben's path, as well as accept that he can no longer be part of mine. How ironic that just as he is ready to go his own way, just when we would have the most to share, Bly believes we need a "break" from each other.

MARRIAGE

In the Iron John world, after adolescent separation has been accomplished, the parents show up next when the son is about to be married. In the story, this is a heterosexual marriage, and though the mother and father are there, they had "given up hope that they would ever see their dear son again." In fact, though they see him, it is not at all clear whether they will ever have a chance to know him again.

The separation process envisioned by Bly interrupts the relationship between the boy and his parents, most especially his mother. Bly implies that the mother's "possessiveness" makes this necessary. However, I glimpse another reason at the wedding, a reason based on another faulty assumption. At her son's wedding, the mother becomes a mother-in-law to his wife. Rather than seeing the addition of a role as leading to the mother's renewed significance to the couple, Bly considers her once central role as the mother of a young son as peripheral now that she is both mother and mother-in-law. It is as if Bly believes that only with distance can the new wife protect her claims on her husband from his mother's clutches.

Here again, the geographic metaphor obscures. For though the mother may no longer be central, it is not distance that will effectively separate mother and son, though it may contribute. Instead, distance will set in if they fail to keep each other apprised of the central experiences in each other's lives. Distance will dominate if they fail to maintain regular contact, in which they invite each other to share in meaningful ways in their lives.

A son will usually choose to share less with his mother once he has a loving partner. A mother, though aware of the loss, can usually feel content about it if she is assured of some intimacy.

The issue is not how frequently they are in contact, but what the contact is like when they have it. Is it intimate or nonintimate? To be intimate, the mother would have to respect that her son is in a primary relationship with his wife. His partner needs to feel assured that the mother's desire for continued contact with her son will not thwart her, or interfere with her relationship to her husband. This can be done. Moreover, mothers-in-law can have relationships with their daughters-in-law that allow three-way intimacy to emerge.

I know that this is the case. As a wife I have been doubly blessed with knowing two mothers-in-law: my mother, who loved Hilary with the fierce passion and interest she applied to me, and Hilary's mother, who made room for me in her relationship with Hilary even as we forged our own connection. These threesomes made me know that there is another version of mother-in-law, one compatible with the version of mother I have been at pains to describe.

In the Iron John world neither the mother nor the mother-in-law is seen as she is or can be, but only as the boy fears she may be. He doesn't recognize her, because there has been no ongoing process by which he has been taught to know the mother as a person in her own right. This is the process I have tried to build jointly with my children, a process of mutual knowing.

Separation as Mutual Knowing, Not (Only) Independence

Naming adolescence as a phase in which parents and children, mother and adolescent son and daughter, are freer to know each other will strike many people as odd. I am mindful that my ideas are provisional—after all, my oldest child is only seventeen. So I draw on other sources too: my clinical work, memories of my own youth, and conversations with other parents and teenagers, always seeing my ideas as tentative and this writing as a report from the front. Accordingly, I have become very observant of and curious about adolescents and their parents, about what they do and also about their theories regarding why. Naturally, I include myself in this scrutiny.

Two years ago, following a lovely, cozy morning with Miranda, then nearly twelve, I drove her to school with a good friend of mine who was visiting from New York. After we dropped Miranda off, I turned to my friend and said, "These are precious days. I know it can't last." The mother of a grown daughter and son herself, my friend said, "It returns." To which I replied, "I know. I don't know why I said that. I know it doesn't vanish forever or entirely. I really don't know why I said what I did."

Then she and I went on through our very busy day, and I didn't give our exchange a second thought. Several hours later, alone, I picked up Miranda from her after-school program. As she got into the car, she began singing a few lines from *The Sound of Music,* "Just wait a year or two. . . ."

"Why are you singing that?" I asked her in a friendly, curious way.

"Because I know I'm going to be an adolescent soon," she replied.

"And what will that mean?" I asked her.

"Then we'll fight all the time," she answered.

Now where could she have gotten that idea? Where did I? If adolescence had a public relations staff, I would have to say it has done a remarkable job of creating a relatively uniform perception of its product. Adolescence is seen by most parents as a difficult stage, and most young adolescents behave as if they have read the same ad copy: they show defiance, anger, irritability, impatience; they withdraw; they criticize. Though often only a short phase, sometimes it lasts for seemingly interminably and unendurably long periods of time. Recognizing shades of my immediately post-treatment self in some of Ben's outbursts, I wondered whether adolescents think, as I did, that separation may overtake them before they are ready for it. Do some teenagers feel that they are being pushed to grow up, be independent, or leave home before they are ready and react accordingly? Does the behavior parents dread signal the child's protest: "Wait, I'm angry about this"?

A few months ago, Miranda volunteered some information on just this theme. She had been particularly difficult the few days before, and she and I were at each other's throats. I wanted her to act more independently, and she wanted more attention, guidance, and support than I wanted to provide. This evening, I was driving her to the library, and trying to discuss with her why she was "resisting" growing up. She was very clear.

"I don't want to grow up and be angry at you and not be close to you anymore."

"Why would your doing more for yourself make us less close?" I asked.

It was a foggy night, and I had pulled the car into the parking lot. The headlights were illuminating water-laden air, and I could see the fog clearly, though not the cars parked several rows ahead. The reversal of figure and ground was pleasing.

Miranda answered deliberately. "The older I get, the more I have to be on my own, without you, and I'm not ready."

"Oh, I know just what you're talking about!" I said. "That's what so many people say about adolescence, but it doesn't have to be what we do. Independence doesn't have to mean that teenagers can't be 'close' to their parents and still think their own ways. I'm not saying that things won't change between us if you do more for yourself, if you become more independent, but, if anything, they will change for the better. We'll have more time to be close in other ways, maybe even more fun ways, if I'm not spending my time doing tasks that you can do. In our family, growing up does not have to mean growing apart."

I think we were both enormously relieved by that brief conversation. Understanding the significance of her behavior differently, I changed my way of handling her sometimes irritatingly childish episodes, and she, lo and behold, stopped the behavior. The conversation and its aftermath dissolved the negative cycle we were in. Too, it emboldened me to think that I was on the right track toward extending my ideas about intimacy to adolescent separation.

One month away from her thirteenth birthday, Miranda was feeling concern precisely about a failure of intimacy: she worried that adolescence would deprive her of intimate conversation with me. She feared that either she or I would withdraw from the other. Our conversation made me think about my clinical work with adolescents. Typically, adolescents and their families come to therapists with problems that appear to concern the teenager's wanting more independence than the parents are prepared to give. Yet this almost invariably covers more troubling, often less accessible, issues. In reviewing my adolescent family cases, I was struck by how often our work had shifted over time from issues of independence to misunderstanding. I often started with angry, disaffected teenagers and their angry, frustrated parents, and ended with parents and children engaged in substantive, if painful, talk with each other. While the adolescent may have started our work together complaining about rules and limits, she often shifted to revealing great sadness at feeling misunderstood or not understood.

Work with sixteen-year-old Lynn and her mother, Audrey, had fit this sequence. As a family therapist, I routinely see adolescents with their parents or families, and only after I have a clear idea of the issues do I consider whom I will see, in what combinations. Initially, I often meet with the member of the family who is most willing to come; that was Audrey. "Therapy is stupid!" Lynn had informed her mother. "If you want to go, that's your business, but I'm not going."

Audrey, a single parent of two adolescents, was deeply discouraged and enraged. She had a long list of complaints and worries about Lynn, who she feared was throwing away her life on the wrong friends and the wrong activities. She feared for her physical safety most of all. After talking with her, I asked her to invite Lynn to come to a single session that would be conjoint: that is, I would see the two women together but with no expectations of what, if anything, our next steps might be.

A sullen, hostile, flamboyantly dressed Lynn arrived for the appointment and grimly sat on the couch next to her mother. Although I had offered to arrange the appointment directly with her, she had acquiesced to her mother's request that she attend once but hadn't wanted to speak to me on the phone. The meeting was alternately tense and explosive. Lynn and Audrey often had diametrically opposing views of their situation, and both were extremely hurt by, as well as furious with, the other. In my experience, the work with a parent-child pair is often remarkably similar to the painstaking work I do with couples. I identify the different beliefs each has about those situations—trivial or significant—that recurrently lead to conflict between them. Sitting with Lynn and Audrey felt much like sitting with an estranged couple, only they, like other parent-child, mother-daughter pairs, could never truly be free of each other, even if they never saw each other again. Their motivation to work things out, though strained and not readily available, was latent. They needed some success in their relationship. They needed to have a single experience of agreement or mutual acknowledgment to instill hope that a therapeutic enterprise could repair the mess they were in with each other.

I tried what I always try first, which is to ask each person to describe the current conflicts from her point of view. Usually people can manage this format, though it requires that each person listen while the other speaks. Lynn and Audrey could not. Each constantly interrupted the other, attacking or accusing the other of lying. Instead, I shifted formats and said I would interview each in the presence of the other, Lynn first. I gave Audrey paper and a pen and asked her to make notes, as if she were behind a one-way mirror.

Lynn's initial story hinged on the fact that her mother didn't trust her. "She doesn't trust me, so it doesn't matter anymore what I do. Why should I do what she wants me to do if she won't believe me anyway?" I asked her to talk about what it was like in the present, and then move to her thoughts about the history of her idea that her mother didn't trust her. When did it start to be like this? Why?

Lynn was definite. "From the beginning. She's never trusted me. Even though I'm the oldest, she's always trusted my brother more. She thinks I'm stupid. She always has. There's nothing I'll ever be able to do to change her mind."

Her last sentence was not said with rage alone. I glanced over to see if Audrey had noticed the pain and poignancy in Lynn's voice, but her face was buried in the pad, and she was writing notes, seemingly unaware that the conversation had paused while we looked toward her. The moment was an opening for me. I wanted to create a space for Lynn to talk about herself in such a way that her pain would be more prominent in her story than blame. I wanted Audrey to hear Lynn's unhappiness, to banish the monolithic impression Audrey had that Lynn cared for nothing and nobody. I wanted to help Lynn tell a story that could arouse in her mother emotions distinct from the ones that had surfaced in reaction to the kind of talking they had been doing.

I was only partly successful. Lynn told a story that I found very compelling, but when they traded places and I asked Audrey to reflect on what she had heard, she felt blamed and, therefore, she retaliated. Later, when Audrey added a bit of context to Lynn's story that Lynn could not have known, Lynn clearly became interested, though she, too, largely just took notes while her mother spoke.

Audrey felt hopeless, guilty, and angry in seemingly equal measure. She wanted Lynn to understand how hard her life had been, but Lynn had heard this too many times to notice whether or not her mother was talking about her experience in any new ways. Lynn's listening was on automatic pilot. Both women, actually, looked incredibly bored as Audrey talked about the travails of being a single parent.

Through my questioning, I tried to maneuver Audrey into unknown territory, into talking about something she had never said out loud, much less to Lynn. I asked her whether her parents trusted her, and this question interested them both. Lynn stopped writing. Audrey talked about how burdened she felt as the eldest child in her family—her mother's confidante about the family's financial worries, her father's confidante about his marital infidelities. "Yes, my parents trusted me, but maybe that wasn't so great either!"

Although the discussion lasted no more than three or four minutes, we were able to talk about the different meanings trust had for Audrey and Lynn. It was a brief episode in a generally rancorous session, but an important one. Momentarily, they saw each other with fresh eyes and heard each other newly. They could not impose meaning on each other, for they were struggling to render their own thoughts about this topic. They also listened to each other. In a wildly stormy relationship, an intimate interchange happened.

As a therapist, these are the moments I am trying to facilitate. Out of just such moments, tattered relationships get woven back together, as Lynn's and Audrey's did. I saw them together twelve times over a six-month period. Unlike many therapists who work with adolescents, I assumed that their talking together would be helpful. I did see Lynn privately when she requested it, and I did keep confidential those matters she asked me to, within the guidelines that the three of us worked out in advance. Audrey didn't believe that she needed to know everything, except when safety was an issue. Lynn understood this concern, in her own way. "What do you think, that I'm an idiot? That I want to do something stupid and die?"

The battles over what Lynn did gradually gave way to conversations about who each of these women were: what they thought, felt, liked, and disliked. They had great passions and great strengths, including considerable comfort with expressing anger.

They left having reestablished a way to feel intimate with one another. Each was more equipped, though not perfectly or infallibly so, to tolerate not understanding the other in order more fully to understand her. "The birth of dialogue," as Z. D. Gurevitch says, "is contingent on the emergence of otherness." I did not assume that in order for Lynn to become independent she had to distance herself from her mother. Quite the contrary: I believed that she would feel more able to work toward independence if she and her mother were more known to each other.

Carol Gilligan and her colleagues at the Harvard Project for the Psychology of Women and the Development of Girls say that girls take their feelings and thoughts "out of relationship" during adolescence because they can see that they are "denied and denigrated by powerful adults, ignored or glossed over or trivialized by cultural conventions and knowledge." In the work that I do, as a therapist and a mother, I am proposing that a mother can be her daughter's ally in opposing, together, the problem for which the solution is removing oneself from the relationship.

Lynn and her mother put themselves back into relationship with each other. They left feeling "close," a culturally sanctioned if culturally idealized way for a mother and daughter to feel about each other. Adolescent sons and mothers are less fortunate, because the culture does not encourage their "closeness." In Euripides' *Orestes,* the young Orestes kills his mother in an act that signifies his extinguishing her influence on him. Does a mother, having internalized this cultural message, collude with it, concurring in some fundamental way that she is bad for her son and thus acquiescing in the culture's efforts to alienate her from him? And what of the correspondingly fierce pressure on a boy to avoid the appearance of being close to his mother, of being a "mama's boy"? Some sons seek a geographic solution to the "problem" of continuing a relationship with their mothers as they get older.

When my son Ben was an infant, I read Feenie Ziner's account of joining *her* son Ben in British Columbia in *Within This Wilderness: The True Story of a Mother's Journey to Rediscover Her Son.* I was extraordinarily moved by the book, making a mental note to reread it when my little one grew up and left home.

In her autobiographical narrative, Ziner describes her literal and metaphoric journey to rediscover her son, who is living alone on a remote Canadian lake in the most primitive conditions. On this journey, she must reattach herself to him, distinguish the messages from him that are about desiring connection. The book is a stunning unfolding of Ziner's slow appreciation that her son, though he has put as much distance as he can

between himself and his family, does not now desire psychological distance. He invites his mother to know him, and he opens
himself to knowing her—a little more than ever before.

She is primed to interpret him as wanting distance. Each
teaches the other that this does not have to be so. At first, Ziner
experiences her son as devaluing her.

" '. . . I just don't understand where you get the fortitude!' I
said.

"He didn't reply at once, but when I looked at his face it had
suddenly gone soft. His eyes were lustrous, brimming. 'Don't
you, Mom? Don't you, really?' he asked."

At this stage in their journey, she does not understand that
this is the best he can do to express his longing for and appreciation of his mother. Neither of them has the idea that they can
find ways of respectfully being intimate with each other, even if
intermittently.

By the end of the book, they have invented this idea together.
For the mother it means moving through "the pause" of recognizing difference and believing that she is good for her son and
of value to him. For Ben it means letting her know that he has
prepared a place for her in his heart. Ben takes his mother to a
giant tree in a remote corner of the forest in which he lives, and
there she climbs up "three rough, ax-hewn steps. . . . It was hol-
low and huge, its core blackened by fire. . . . As my eyes grew
accustomed to the darkness, I discerned a figure scratched upon
the inner surface of the wood—the figure of a man falling head-
long through space. I did not know who put it here. It could
have been an Indian sign, or it could have been Ben's own draw-
ing, his self-portrait.

" 'No,' I thought. 'I cannot leave it at that.'

"There was another truth, and it was just as holy as the truth
inscribed upon the walls. It was a human truth that had to be
asserted in the face of terrible and pitiless gods.

"It was not enough to witness the sign. I had to alter it. . . .
Ben was part of my life, and what connected us to one another
was stronger than what separated us. We were all fallen angels;
our redemption lay in the lives we shared with one another.

"The fingers in my pocket curled around chalk. I took it out and drew another falling figure alongside the first, linking their hands. And then another, and another, until I covered the blackened walls with a circle of angels, an ongoing wheel of life. . . .

" 'It's my message, Ben,' I said.

"We wept in one another's arms. . . ."

They leave the tree, and later look back at it. But hers is not the final word.

" 'Do you see these steps?' he said when I reached the rock ledge.

" 'Yes . . .'

" 'I cut those steps for you, more than two years ago. I knew, then, that you would come.' "

This is the last line in the book. He knew she would come. We live in a culture in which our ideas about the mother-son relationship leave sons waiting for their mothers in literal or figurative remote places. As a mother, I must resist this idea and insist that mutual knowing is my son's birthright as much as my daughter's.

The opportunities for practicing mutual knowing do not always declare themselves obviously. This spring, some time before Hilary and I were planning to go away for a weekend, I told the children to make arrangements for themselves to stay at friends' houses while we were gone. Ben asked to stay at our house, and I told him he could not. A few weeks later, he brought up the subject again. This time he said he felt I didn't trust him. I was relieved that he had told me, because I had been annoyed about his procrastination in arranging a plan for himself. Here was his reason. I tried to explain myself to him.

"This is not a decision about you, but about me. I have decided I don't want to worry while I am away. I'm involved with issues about loss that make me worry about your safety, and this is not a safe world. I understand that it is my task to handle my fears, but this is not a weekend I want to work on them. This is my vacation, and I want to know that you are with adults who are watching out for you. I need you to believe that this is about

me and the world we live in, not you. You live in an environment and I'm worried about that place, not about you."

I then went on to identify some of the reasons I think I have
issues with loss, a history he is not unfamiliar with, but which
is not one I had yet summarized for him. I linked my mother's
death, his and Miranda's early medical problems, and my cancer
into a story about my sensitivity to and worry about loss. I believed that telling him about myself was appropriate and that
asking him to accommodate to my need in this instance was fair.
I did not believe that I was burdening him beyond what he could
be reasonably expected to bear. I was not asking him to help me
with my issues about loss, but to use the information as background for understanding what he felt was an irrational and
overprotective decision.

For me, this talk with Ben is symbolic of the changes I have
made. I had to move from silence to speech. I have done this
work. I can imagine, however, a future in which my challenge
will be with what I wish to keep private, rather than what I want
to share. For now, I am saying more than I ventured to do in
the past. Ben listened and reluctantly accepted my verdict about
the weekend, making it clear that he wished I would change. He
did not bring it up again. I felt respected by him, and, frankly,
incredibly appreciative.

He let me tell him about myself, just as I have let him tell me
about himself. Learning about each other is quintessentially mutual work, and we teach each other how to do it. It is also a step
that some mothers and their children may wait too long to take.
During the car ride when Miranda stopped playing the tape of
Les Misérables and we talked about whether or not Hilary alone
would love her in the way she needed, we also talked about what
my cancer had meant to her. I was braced to hear many awful
meanings, none of which prepared me for what she finally said.

"I think I learned how much I love you, and now I have trouble getting angry at you," she volunteered. We talked some
more. Though she could not have formulated her problem quite
like this, I think she also meant, "I think I learned how much I
love you too young." She seemed to be saying to me that I had

become a person to her, a person in my own right, not just an extension of her, there to gratify, educate, love, and keep safe.

Her comment made my head spin. First, I was extraordinarily relieved that she hadn't pulled back from me—my trick—to protect herself from possible loss. Second, I felt certain that time would take care of her expression of anger: she had passionate feelings all the time, and we were heading into adolescence. Finally, I thought, she has had a glimpse of the reality children in other cultures see even earlier. If anything, I speculated that our relationship would benefit from her really seeing me, knowing I am vulnerable, too.

African-American women have written about this aspect of their relationship with their mothers. Many of them have specifically attributed the evolutionary, not revolutionary, quality of their separation from their mothers as attributable to the fact that racism forces them to see early the actuality of their mothers' lives and the realities of their mothers as human beings. Perhaps, too, because both mother and daughter know that the oppression they experience within their own relationship is secondary to the vaster oppression within which they both live, African-American daughters and mothers begin the process of knowing each other earlier.

How this knowledge fares is another story. Whether any mother and daughter are able to fully engage in the often tedious process of listening, correcting, and challenging the other in order to achieve a more accurate and complete image is a dilemma in any culture.

Miranda and I, Ben and I, are on our way. Miranda is highly sensitive to the wider oppression that now hovers over her life— the weight that fear of my premature death creates for her, and for me. Ben seems to sequester his awareness of my cancer, rarely mentioning it. Our process of mutual knowing does not feel, as it does with Miranda, that it has had a supercharged boost from this other realm. He is hardly blasé about my illness, however. "Mom, if you die," he has said, "it will be the worst thing that ever happened in my life. But right now you're all right, and I don't have to think about it." Which is just fine.

Fine, that is, as long as he can think enough about it to take me in the way I really am—a person periodically more worried, more frightened, more sober than I would probably otherwise be.

Separation as Loss

In addition to independence and mutual knowing, separation means loss. When teenagers leave home, their departure is clearly a loss. They aren't there to nudge you, eat with you, talk on the phone, leave their things around, play their music, take care of the animals, hug you, bring over their friends, do errands, leave out the milk . . . in short, share your daily life. But, as I have said, this loss is counterbalanced in my mind by addition. As they move out in the world, their expanding lives add dimension to the lives of the people who cannot go with them but can be enriched by them. I anticipate a bittersweet time.

Not all separations are bittersweet; some are bitter. Children who leave and don't come back; children who withdraw from their parents' lives and refrain from all but the most meager sharing; children who follow paths that their parents are unable to acknowledge or accept; children who live violent lives—all these create separations from their parents that are painful and unrelentingly bleak. I feel enormous compassion for these kinds of separations.

Death is another kind of separation, one that is also characterized by loss, not addition. My mother and I separated twice; my children and I not once yet. Each of my partings from my mother has taught me something of lasting value—perhaps the same thing. With neither separation did I feel that I knew what my mother felt. At the brink of each, she withdrew her vital presence, her voice, and, though she listened to me with her extraordinary intensity, I could not get her to speak.

I never knew just how she felt before I left home for college, because, she later told me, she could not imagine my understanding what she had to tell me. Had she told me then, she would have said that she was of two minds about my leaving: sad and ecstatic. She was sad because she would see me less;

ecstatic because she could write without a hovering consciousness of me. She was right that I would have been taken aback, hurt, perhaps even angry. I certainly would not have understood—immediately, that is.

I would not have understood because I hadn't been a mother yet. In order to understand, she would have needed to take me along with her, into her experiences, to allow me to grasp empathically what I could not grasp automatically. It would have taken time and work, intimate work. We could have done it.

The next time we separated, she was dying. Perhaps because I was in Boston, confined by my pregnancy to telephone calls, she stopped sharing as much of her experience as she had before her disease moved from chronic to terminal. Painfully, as she neared her end, she withdrew from the mutual knowing that in her final years had made our relationship so special. She was as curious as ever about me, but her thoughts and her feelings receded, thinning as rapidly as her wasting body.

Being with her then was as painful as it was precious. Not only because of the imminence of her physical departure from this earth, but because she had departed from me in other ways as well. She no longer spoke about her dying, for instance. Nor was it clear to either me or anyone else in my family that she believed she was dying. In some way that I still don't understand, for reasons that I continue to puzzle about, none of us was able to share her approaching experience of death with her. I have never felt so lonely in my life.

My father, my sister, and I stayed with my mother from the first hours of her last hospitalization until they took her body away. She was fully engaged with us until moments before she lost consciousness; she died several hours later. She talked to each of us, and to all of us. I managed to tell her what I needed her to know, without saying good-bye. So did we all. I held her hand, stroked her, watched her dissolve as she was eaten by the cancer within, and I was totally unprepared for her final words.

Though private, they have been printed already, added to my mother's book *Intimations of Mortality,* which was published posthumously. Her last words were: "Forgive me, but this is absurd."

Probably no words have preoccupied me more than these. Try as I might, I have been unable to understand how at the moment of death, she—she of all people—could have said "Forgive me."

Only she, of course, could help me to understand. I would have to say that the work this book records has been, in part, my effort to ensure that I will never say "forgive" if I mean "farewell." Pondering her words has helped me to change, though. Before my cancer was diagnosed, I could not imagine a way out of the dilemma I experienced on the beach—that moment when I feared that the very detachment I would need to get through dying would be the quality most hurtful to my children. Thinking about my mother's death, thinking about mine, I have seen that conversation with my children could dissolve that conflict. We would have to talk.

In my view, now, I see separation as that time in family life when mutual knowing becomes possible—when it can begin. Whether this is at age two or five or ten or fifteen or thirty will depend on a myriad of factors. Whenever it is, separation will be about voice and listening. For through listening to each other well, avidly, and devotedly, we draw out voice and accompany each other on our separate journeys. Separation is not the beginning of distance but the opportunity for another kind of closeness.

TEN

Challenging Cultural Beliefs Together

Radical Listening

When sons or daughters listen to their mother so that she is able to know, articulate, and share her thoughts and feelings, they are challenging cultural beliefs. It is a form of practicing cultural resistance. When a mother invites her older children to share their evolving life stories with her, and they, feeling her nonintrusive respect, do so, they are practicing cultural resistance. They are resisting countervailing cultural pressures that confuse intimacy with intrusion and assume that the natural course of development is separation, not complexity. They are living a partnership model in a family.

Why use the term cultural resistance? Cultural resistance, first and foremost, is a challenge to ourselves. It requires a willingness to turn the countless messages we receive and produce daily, each with its embedded directives for thinking, feeling, and action, into the stuff of consciousness. It requires radical alertness to listen for that which we are not meant to hear, and to see that which we are not meant to see. Cultural resistance makes the invisible, visible; the silent, heard. Further, it means accepting that we are not by nature free of cultural influences, but social from the start. Turning to our *own* experience to learn what we *really* think and feel may prove an untrustworthy guide, since we will find in ourselves the same cultural messages that we can, with practice, identify outside ourselves. Even the body sends no direct signal that isn't interpreted by a perceptual and conceptual apparatus honed by living with others who have learned from their cultures what these supposedly "neutral" body signals mean. If we are going to learn what truly suits us, and not just what the cultures we live in have convinced us we should desire, we are going to have to use more critical thinking about our cultural context, be more open to diverse others, and add a lively imagination to routine introspection.

If cultural resistance is preeminently personal, it is also social. Mothers are ideally suited to marshal resistance, because they are on the front lines of the cultural transmission that takes place in families. Precisely because families are the ideal sites for indoctrination, families, of whatever type, are perfect for resistance too. But they pose particular challenges. If we resist received ideas, we are likely to develop a wider range of ideas and values. With variation, differences among family members will widen, not narrow. Consensus, so often favored as the means to rapport, will be harder to achieve. Instead, families will have to find ways of creating harmony from diversity.

Within families, as any mother—and any family therapist— will attest, listening to each other is the heart of the matter. In most cultures there is the expectation that mothers will listen. The idealized mother is a person who listens and absorbs the troubles of her mate and children; a person whose listening soothes. I am proposing that this kind of listening be shared in families—that partners and children, too, listen to the voice of the mother. As Sara Ruddick has said, listening, really listening, to the voices of mothers "could be considered a form of resistance."

But more than that, I am proposing that all family members listen to each other. I am proposing that listening well to others, not imposing meaning, be a regular practice—in families and elsewhere. Helping a voice to be heard is truly radical listening.

Families can also be the place to start transforming, not reproducing, the cultural messages we are exposed to so relentlessly that we internalize them. We must listen to *messages* with which, like air, we are surrounded. We must try to decode meaning: symbols, gestures, and words. Hear words: single ones, groups of them, words in anecdotes and stories. By resisting words, resisting ideas, resisting what we read, we will be practicing cultural resistance. Feeling firmly connected to others provides a safe foundation to challenge the cultural messages that oppress us both as family members and as citizens. Families can and, I believe, must talk with each other about issues such as racism, sexism, ethnic and religious prejudice, poverty, homophobia, consumerism, violence, global destruction, and human-rights violations. These are the issues that make up the family's environment and are as vital to its integrity as what happens "within."

Where I Am in the Journey Now

People often ask me whether having cancer has changed my life. The question maddens me, for, literalist that I am, the form of the question always makes me think that cancer is being given credit for some good when, in my estimation, cancer has been responsible for only ill. I, on the other hand, have made the best I could of having had breast cancer when I did.

I have had some formidable allies. I cannot imagine going through this experience without my family. My children have suffered worries I wish they didn't have, but throughout they have remained lovingly connected to me. Hilary has cared for me physically, emotionally, and spiritually. Though this was no surprise, it remains a gift of inestimable value. He has been with me not just in the middle of the night, but all through the night.

My parents provide continuous inspiration. My father, who has had health troubles of his own, has been consistently upbeat with me. Toward the end of my chemotherapy, anticipating the resources I would need and knowing where to find them, I wrote to my father. I asked him if he would talk with me about how he managed to live each day with uncertainty, and how he managed to live life so fully despite it. He called me within hours of receiving his mail.

"I'm flattered by your letter," he said, "but I don't know what you're talking about. What uncertainty?"

"That's what I mean, Dad. I need some of that attitude. How do you manage to keep your fears at bay?" I replied.

"Look," he said, making his voice low and direct. "I set myself short-term goals. I keep my eye on the future. My short-term goal is to dance with you at Miranda's wedding."

My mother had short- and long-term goals. She wrote in her journal until three months before she died. One of the last phone calls she made was to her editor to inform him that her next book project was going to be a story for children about grand-mothers. She remained indomitable, loving, and open until the last hours of her life. Near the end, on one clear, still night, she walked outside, hitched to her oxygen tank, and asked us to watch the moon with her. Hugging her sweet, emaciated body, I found that her joy pushed my pain aside. I looked up with her in awe at a universe that offered such perfect comfort in the midst of infinitesimally small dramas. She never saw the moon again.

When I was a child, my mother talked of seeing the year 2000. She would say, "I hope to be alive for the second millennium." When she first said that, I quickly did the arithmetic and I remember thinking, Very likely, very likely. Privately, I have started to think that I would like to see the second millennium. My children will be nearly old enough for me to feel safe. Very likely, very likely.

In the meantime, I must try to make myself feel safe. I do this in many ways, one of which is to resist the meaning of cancer itself. Cancer is a disease that is diagnosed by people sitting in a lab deciding whether this cell or that looks like this cell or that. Having cancer is not definitive. People make a judgment. I had cancer, the disease. But the experience of cancer is also a story like any other. It is as shareable as sadness, and its moods are as amenable to shifts as are those of sadness. I asked my family and friends to let me share cancer with them. In doing so, they agreed to have a little bit of cancer too—the way it makes you vulnerable; the way it makes you grateful. Though my body contained the cancer cells, a community of concern contained the meaning of the cancer. When I had more cancer than most, they did, too, and now that I have none, they live cancer-free. Friends, extended family, and colleagues have all been wonderful; I have known definitively that people want me to live.

I have also tried to understand the context of the cancer itself. I do try to eat well, exercise, avoid stress, and respond early to my body's signals. Additionally, I am interested in the political context of this particular cancer. Balancing my political commitment with my emotional capacities to handle the onerous facts, I protest the lack of attention that this disease has received in the government's funding of cancer research. I support wholeheartedly the political critique made by women's health-care groups about the status of breast cancer research, treatment, and prevention.

My relationship to cancer is ongoing. I get routine monitoring, which is a blessing and a curse. Times when there is "concern" from the doctor are very challenging for me. Worried about overburdening my family and friends, knowing how scary it can be, I sometimes pull my sails down in the wind, as it were, preferring to let the puff pass by rather than have my sails luffing away, signaling distress to those nearby. I am still trying to figure out whom this tack is for, me or others.

Though I sometimes pull away from my nonmedical community, I am never alone, because my medical community is always available. I wish I did not have to have these ongoing relationships. I also know things now that I would have preferred never to know, or to know later.

My doctors have been, without exception, wonderful. Each has been willing to enter my kind of conversation, understanding that talk can "heal" some of the places where cancer lurks. It can heal scary thoughts. For instance, when I began writing this book, my elation was balanced by my fear about the harm I might do, since I awoke spontaneously to write at 4:30 in the morning. My oncologist said the right words at the critical moment: "How do you know it's not more stressful not to write a book that is in you than to get too little sleep?" Could this book have been written without that encouragement?

I think less about death than I did in 1989, the year of my diagnosis, but I think about it more than I would like. I tend to be a planner. I also take umbrage when others talk about death in ways that contradict what I have come to understand. When Barbara Bush spoke to the graduating class at Wellesley College in May of 1990, she said, "At the end of your life, you will never regret not having passed one more test, not winning one more verdict or not closing one more deal. You will regret time not spent with a husband, a friend, a child, or a parent." The sentiment enraged me. Who is the "you" she is referring to? I thought. At the end of one's life, I imagine, contrary to what Mrs. Bush said, one regrets what one hasn't gotten a chance to do—all the pieces of a life that didn't make it into the quilt. The people Mrs. Bush is talking about who regretted time not spent with family and friends are people who dropped intimate connection from the fabric of their lives so that, at the end, rightly, they are sad.

My mother devoted her best years and the majority of her waking hours to her intimate relationships with her children and husband, parents, friends, and extended family. At the end of her life, she regretted what she had had too little of—not love, but work. She regretted that she wouldn't get to write another book.

If one is full of life, one will have regrets at the end of life. It seems to me that this is inevitable. Still, I am writing now, because I do not want to have regrets about this later. Nor do I want to regret missed opportunities for intimate connection. This book expresses what is, has been, and can be heard in the many relationships I have.

When I began treatment, the image I used was that of a quilt, the common, every-woman-uses-it image, "quilt." I would say to myself, I—quiltmaker—have been handed some pieces I would not have chosen. They are not the shape, the color, the texture, the design I would have selected for my quilt, my life. But I do not get to choose the pieces, just the composition.

I have tried to stitch together the pieces of my life—the ones I have chosen, the ones I have adopted, the ones I have been given, the ones I have made, and the ones I have been dealt— into the most durable cloth I can. I have striven for a quilt that is serviceable to me and to others, many others. There are moments when I try to stitch with artistry, but more often I try to stitch thoughtfully and honestly. It's my best bet.

This book is of a piece. It has been stitched, like all the other pieces of my life, in conversation with others. Together we have fashioned an account with which we can live.

APPENDIX

Questions to Consider

Though I have written the following questions and suggestions from the perspective of a mother, they can be adapted for use by other family members.

1. Imagine that you can make transparent the beliefs that underlie your feelings, thoughts, and actions. What are they? Record daily events that seem rich or complex in meaning. Try to understand the ideas and values that your way of participating in these events represents. Share this work with a trusted person. Perhaps encourage a friend to work on this as a project simultaneously, so that you can compare and contrast what you are each learning.

2. Consider whether or not, or under what circumstances, you tell others what you really experience as a mother. If you do not tell, or feel that you cannot, what circumstances prevent you from doing so? What would have to change to make this pattern different? Whom would you select to see, if he or she could truly listen to your mother's voice?

3. Ask yourself what a mother should and should not do. What stories come to mind about a "good" mother and a "bad" mother? Notice whether or not your thinking about mothers is permeated by a good/bad split. If it is, notice the areas that are

coded good or bad. How do you feel and act when you violate your standards for a good mother? If your thinking about motherhood does not include this split, how do you account for your escaping this common, crippling way of thinking?

4. Is it difficult for you to choose whether to do something for yourself or for others? Do you sometimes feel torn between taking care of yourself or attending to someone else? Do you ever feel resentful of others? How do you handle these feelings: by taking care of yourself at all costs; by putting yourself last; or by making situation-specific decisions?

5. What are the stories about yourself that you have assumed were inappropriate to share with your children? What consequences do you feel there have been in your relationships with your children from withholding these stories from them? Can you imagine any benefit to you, to them, or to the relationship of beginning to share more of yourself with them? How can you ensure that sharing will be informative rather than burdensome to them?

6. How would your life change if your workplace truly cared about your family life? What are the ways your employer could make your life easier without unduly inconveniencing others at work or reducing your productivity? Make two lists and prioritize according to the changes that would make the largest difference to you and the least difference to your employer. Select the item on the two lists that feels most worth fighting for in terms of benefit to you and likelihood of success. Talk to co-workers, if you have any, and see if they would support your effort to make a change.

7. Make a list of who does what tasks in your family. Include two categories: who thinks about and plans, takes responsibility for, and remembers; and who does the work. Ask family members to help you generate the list. Notice the distribution of work. If there are inequities, have a conversation about what may produce these inequities. Try to have this conversation in the spirit of curiosity, not blame. Suggest that each family member make one change as an experiment and evaluate its impact

after a week or two. Repeat this process until you are satisfied with your arrangement.

8. What did you learn from your family of origin about being a wife? What has been positive and what has been negative about this learning? Notice whether there are relationships in your life in which you are or feel vulnerable to domination. Do you resist domination? Think about what experiences have caused you to respond as you do. If you think you experience more domination than someone else who had your best interest at heart would approve, what do you think you can safely do to address this circumstance? What might the consequences be if you began making changes? What are the resources in your community for people who are trying to make these kinds of changes? If you are married, how would your relationship with your partner shift if you were to construe yourself as a loving partner, not as a wife?

9. Describe your ideas about the ways a father is important to a family. If your children have or have had a father, describe how you think your family benefits or did benefit from having one. How could you promote what is of value, whether with your children's actual father, a substitute father, an honorary father, or an interested other, male or female?

10. What shifts for you in your thinking about relationships if you conceptualize intimacy as made up of single intimate or nonintimate interactions, each of which can be directly influenced by your behavior? If you believe that a mother can teach her children to recognize whether or not others are imposing meaning on them—verbally or nonverbally—what issues immediately arise for you?

11. If you believe that, over time, it is desirable to stay intimate with a son and that intimacy with a daughter is not automatic, how might you behave with your son and/or daughter now? If you believe that you could retain your position as a respected figure without behaving in an authoritarian way, would you consider sharing more of yourself with your children than you do presently? Would you provide or impose meaning

less? Are you aware when you withdraw from relationships, or reject others' attempts to communicate, and why you do this?

12. What might change in your relationships with your children if you believed that, as they grew older, you were helping them to both know you better and become more independent?

13. What experience do you have with constructively managing diverse opinion? What did you learn in your family of origin about diversity, and how does this learning influence you now?

14. If you asked everyone in your family to take as a goal that the family be a place in which people feel at home, by which I mean that they feel enabled, loved, safe, empowered, and respected, what steps would have to be taken to bring this to pass?

15. Do you think you listen to others in such a way that they truly feel invited to speak? Notice if you are more likely to listen well to one or another family member, and speculate about the reasons for this.

16. Think about these questions in your own sweet time, recognizing that cultural resistance is a process of discovery, commitment, and transformation that cannot be rushed.

NOTES

Chapter One

1   "I think the key . . .": Nancy Mairs, *Carnal Acts* (New York: HarperCollins, 1990), 61.

3   According to the psychologist Jerome Bruner . . . : Jerome Bruner, *Acts of Meaning* (Cambridge, MA.: Harvard University Press, 1990), 77.

9   Voice is a metaphor . . . : See Mary Field Belenky, Blythe McVicker Clinchy, Nancy Rule Goldberger, and Jill Mattuck Tarule, *Women's Ways of Knowing: The Development of Self, Voice, and Mind* (New York: Basic Books, 1986), 18, for a discussion of the metaphor of voice as women use it.

9   "I was trying . . .": Sharon O'Brien, *Willa Cather: The Emerging Voice* (New York: Oxford University Press, 1987), 173.

10   This shift from . . . : I call the coupling of voice with listening the authentication of voice. It differs from validation of voice in that validation depends on the other person's using his or her experience to measure the accuracy of the speaker's communication, whereas authentication requires a willingness to hear fully the speaker's meaning. They are radically different activities.

Chapter Two

16   I have been interested . . . : The theoretical underpinnings of this chapter derive from discourse theory. I have read a variety of papers and books, both primary and secondary sources, that have helped me apply ideas about discourse to my project on mothers' stories. Among them are: Michel Foucault, *Power/Knowledge: Selected Interviews & Other Writings 1972–1977*, ed. by Colin Gordon (New York: Pantheon Books, 1980); Irene Diamond and Lee Quinby, eds., *Feminism and Foucault: Reflections on Resistance* (Boston: Northeastern University Press, 1988); Mary McCanney Gergen, ed., *Feminist Thought and the Structure of Knowledge* (New York: New York University Press, 1988); Rachel T. Hare-Mustin and Jeanne Marechek, eds., *Making a Difference: Psychology and the Construction of Gender* (New Haven: Yale University Press, 1990); Linda J.

Nicholson, *Feminism/Postmodernism* (New York: Routledge, 1990); Michael White and David Epston, *Narrative Means to Therapeutic Ends* (New York: Norton, 1990).

17 During my cancer treatment . . . : See Joan W. Scott, "Deconstructing Equality-Versus-Difference: Or, the Uses of Poststructuralist Theory for Feminism" in Marianne Hirsch and Evelyn Fox Keller, eds., *Conflicts in Feminism* (New York: Routledge, 1990), 135–36.

18 So pervasive was this idea . . . : Susan Sontag, *Illness as Metaphor* (New York: Farrar, Straus & Giroux, 1978), 8.

21 These mechanisms were designed . . . : Scott, ibid., discusses the mechanisms by which dominant ideas circulate in the culture.

22 They had the means . . . : I am grateful to Sara Cobb for suggesting Steven Lukes' *Power: A Radical View* (London: Macmillan Press, 1974) as a source for differentiating kinds of power.

28 A good mother . . . : See Elizabeth Badinter, *Mother Love: Myth & Reality* (New York: Macmillan, 1981).

28 Ruth Block's analysis . . . : Ruth H. Block, "American Feminine Ideals in Transition: The Rise of the Moral Mother, 1785–1815," *Feminist Studies* 4 (2): 101–26 (1978).

29 At that time . . . : See E. Ann Kaplan, "Mothering, Feminism and Representation: The Maternal in Melodrama and the Woman's Film 1910–1940" in Christine Gledhill, ed., *Home Is Where the Heart Is: Studies in Melodrama and the Woman's Film* (London: British Film Institute, 1987), 113–37.

29 The "discovery" of the child . . . : Barbara Ehrenreich and Deirdre English, *For Her Own Good: 150 Years of the Experts' Advice to Women* (Garden City, NY.: Anchor Books, 1979).

29 Images of mothers . . . : Ibid., 116.

29 Though this history . . . : See Patricia Hill Collins, "The Meaning of Motherhood in Black Culture and Black Mother/Daughter Relationships," *Sage* 4 (2): 3–10 (1987) for a discussion of the ways this sequence fits primarily white mothers.

29 The profession of the . . . : Ehrenreich and English, *For Her Own Good,* chap. 6.

29 These experts . . . : Linda Gordon, in *Heroes of Their Own Lives: The Politics of Family Violence* (New York: Viking, 1988), writes that at first the "discourse [of mothers] was not dominated by pediatricians, as it later came to be, but by lay women, influenced by feminism," 33.

29 A first phase . . . : See Lois Braverman, "Beyond the Myth of Motherhood," in Monica McGoldrick, Carol M. Anderson, and Froma Walsh, eds., *Women and Families: A Framework for Family Therapy* (New York: Norton, 1989), 232.

29 In "I Stand Here Ironing" . . . : Tillie Olsen, "I Stand Here Ironing," in *Tell Me a Riddle* (New York: Delta, 1989), 2.

29 Dr. Spock's well-known book . . . : Benjamin Spock, *Baby and Childcare* (New York: Pocket Books, 1946).

30 Nancy Chodorow . . . : Nancy Chodorow and Susan Contratto, "The

Fantasy of the Perfect Mother" in Barrie Thorne with Marilyn Yalom, eds., *Rethinking the Family: Some Feminist Questions* (White Plains, NY: Longman Press, 1982), 67.

30 Chodorow and Contratto note . . . : Ibid., 65.

30 "If mothers have . . .": Ibid., 71.

32 Thus few of us . . . : I am not recommending that one can resist a dominating idea by challenging every interaction that embodies it. I would never myself, for instance, correct a child who had just said he or she loved me by asking that child to be more specific about what qualities he or she loved. On the other hand, as part of a conversation that was more playful, I might well begin a game with a child in which we "played" by naming specific qualities we liked about each other. This teaches particularizing.

32 The way I worked it out . . . : See Patricia Paskowicz, *Absentee Mothers* (Totowa, NJ: Allanheld, Osmun, 1982).

33 It is particularly ironic . . . : Helene Deutsch's *The Psychology of Women,* vol. 2: *Motherhood* (New York: Grune & Stratton, 1945) is a striking example of a mother writing from within her professional discipline seemingly divorced from her knowledge as a "maternal thinker." Adrienne Rich's *Of Woman Born: Motherhood as Experience and Institution* (New York: Norton, 1976) and Sara Ruddick's *Maternal Thinking: Toward a Politics of Peace* (Boston: Beacon, 1989) are examples of ways mothers who are professionals can draw on knowledge from both sources.

34 Asked by the male reporter . . . : Thomas Palmer, "Specialists Say Parents Must Be Told of Abuse Cases," *Boston Globe,* July 15, 1991, 13, 24.

34 In a modest . . . : Valuing insights from the mother's position follows from a particular stance on the production of knowledge. I follow a recent tradition described by Evelyn Fox Keller in *Reflections on Gender and Science* (New Haven: Yale University Press, 1985). Sara Ruddick's *Maternal Thinking* is an eloquent treatise on maternal thinking and the practice that derives from it.

34 The writer Tillie Olsen . . . : Tillie Olsen, *Silences* (New York: Delacorte Press/Seymour Lawrence, 1978), 5–46.

34 Thirty years later . . . : Marianne Hirsch, *The Mother-Daughter Plot: Narrative, Psychoanalysis, Feminism* (Bloomington: Indiana University Press, 1989).

35 It is my hope . . . : Gregory Bateson, *Mind and Nature: A Necessary Unity* (New York: Dutton, 1979).

36 In *The Chalice and the Blade* . . . : Riane Eisler, *The Chalice and the Blade* (New York: HarperCollins, 1988).

37 I look at daily life . . . : Adrienne Rich, "Forward," in Sara Ruddick and Pamela Daniels, eds., *Working It Out: 23 Women Writers, Artists, Scientists, and Scholars Talk about Their Lives and Work* (New York: Pantheon, 1977), xvi.

37 In their quilts . . . : Elsa Barkley Brown, "African-American Women's Quilting: A Framework for Conceptualizing and Teaching African-American Women's History," in Micheline R. Malson, Elizabeth Mudimbe-Boyi, Jean F. O'Barr, and Mary Wyer, eds., *Black Women in America* (Chicago: University of Chicago Press, 1990).

Chapter Three

38   Jane Lazarre, *Worlds Beyond My Control* (New York: Dutton, 1991), 116–17.

40   Sara Ruddick has written . . . : Sara Ruddick, *Maternal Thinking,* 34–37.

41   This kind of power . . . : Ibid., 17.

41   Yet not all children . . . : Jane Taylor McDonnell, "Mothering an Autistic Child: Reclaiming the Voice of the Mother," in Brenda O. Daly and Maureen T. Reddy, *Narrating Mothers: Theorizing Maternal Subjectivities* (Knoxville: University of Tennessee Press, 1991), 58–75.

41   They were based on . . . : Nancy Chodorow and Susan Contratto, "The Fantasy of the Perfect Mother," 71.

41   Neither notion has . . . : See Stella Chess and Alexander Thomas, *Origins and Evolution of Behavior Disorders: From Infancy to Early Adult Life* (Cambridge, MA: Harvard University Press, 1987); Jerome Kagan, *The Nature of the Child* (New York: Basic Books, 1984); Rachel T. Hare-Mustin, "The Problem of Gender in Family Therapy Theory," *Family Process* 26:18, 1987.

42   When the dominant ideology . . . : See Nancy Chodorow and Susan Contratto, "The Fantasy of the Perfect Mother."

42   Although the acceptance . . . : See Gloria I. Joseph in a chapter about the mother-daughter relationship for African-American women in *Common Differences: Conflicts in Black and White Feminist Perspectives* (New York: Anchor Press/Doubleday, 1981), 96. Joseph's writing on African-American mother-daughter relationships is pathbreaking. There is little qualitative, descriptive writing to date about the mother-son relationship in African-American families.

42   African-American communities . . . : See Patricia Hill Collins, "The Meaning of Motherhood in Black Culture," 3–10.

42   In addition, African-American communities . . . : Nancy Boyd-Franklin, *Black Families in Therapy: A Multi-Systems Approach* (New York: Guilford Press, 1989).

43   Autism is generally understood today . . . : See Michael Rutter and Erik Schopler, eds., *Autism: A Reappraisal of Concepts and Treatment* (New York: Plenum Press, 1978).

43   The children's oddities . . . : Subsequent to writing the first draft of this chapter I read Jane Taylor McDonnell's essay "Mothering an Autistic Child: Reclaiming the Voice," in *Narrating Mothers.* I was pleased to find many points of similarity in our thinking, all of which are amplified in more depth in her moving essay. For a contrasting, earlier, and pejorative view of the mother's role in the development of autism, see Bruno Bettelheim's *The Empty Fortress: Infantile Autism and the Development of the Self* (New York: Macmillan, 1967).

43   Sue Miller, in her novel . . . : Sue Miller, *Family Pictures* (New York: HarperPaperbacks, 1990).

44   Until recently, mothers . . . : I am describing father-daughter incest because the blaming of mothers has taken place in this framework. Recent work on sexual abuse has revealed that boys are also victimized sexually and that females perpetrate abuse as well as males. Further, sibling incest, which

can be devastating, takes place between cross-sex and same-sex siblings. See Vernon R. Wiehen with Teresa Herring, *Perilous Rivalry: When Siblings Become Abusive* (Lexington, MA.: D. C. Heath, 1991).

44 In fact, in the circumstances . . . : For evidence of mother-blaming in incest, see Linda Gordon, *Heroes of Their Own Lives;* Nicola Gavey, Joy Florence, Sue Pezaro, and Jan Tan, "Mother-Blaming, the Perfect Alibi: Family Therapy and the Mothers of Incest Survivors," in *Journal of Feminist Family Therapy* 2(1): 1–25 (1990); and Janet Liebman Jacobs, "Reassessing Mother Blame in Incest," in Jean F. O'Barr, Deborah Pope, and Mary Wyer, eds., *Ties That Bind: Essays on Mothering and Patriarchy* (Chicago: University of Chicago Press, 1990), 273–87.

44 Having learned to appreciate . . . : See Judith Lewis Herman, *Father-Daughter Incest* (Cambridge, MA: Harvard University Press, 1981) and *Trauma and Recovery: The Aftermath of Violence—from Domestic Abuse to Political Terror* (New York: Basic Books, 1992). However, it is essential that we not replace one dominant explanation—mothers of children who have been incestuously abused are selfish and bad—with another falsifying generalization, that, for instance, they are always blameless. Mothers' reactions to incest are highly variable. Some mothers are devastated for their children. Some refuse to believe their children and support the abuser instead. A mother's response is always complicated, connected to her own history of abuse, history with the abuser, cultural and familial context, and issues of emotional and economic dependence. We might prefer mothers to respond selflessly and devote themselves solely to their children's recovery, but mothers also have their own recovery to attend to when their children have been victimized. Incest creates at least two victims who must become survivors; theories and treatment programs that cannot account for this erase maternal subjectivity. Additionally, in the field of incest the dominant idea that males are perpetrators and females are victims marginalizes the experiences of male survivors and renders female, especially maternal, perpetrators invisible. This has caused indescribable pain to many whose experiences have not been allowed to count.

44 We can imagine . . . : Carolyn Moore Newberger, Isabelle M. Gremy, Christine M. Waternaux, Eli H. Newberger, "Mothers of Sexually Abused Children: Trauma and Repair in Longitudinal Perspective," *American Journal of Orthopsychiatry,* 63:92–102 (1993); Eli H. Newberger, Carolyn Moore Newberger, and Isabelle Gremy, "Dual Vulnerability of Sexually Victimized Mothers and Sexually Victimized Children: A Longitudinal Study," unpublished paper available from the first author, Children's Hospital, 300 Longwood Ave., Boston, MA 02115.

45 Soon, more nonfiction accounts . . . : Two books available that feature the writings of mothers of incest victims are: Sandi Ashley, *The Missing Voice: Writings by Mothers of Incest Victims* (Dubuque, IA: Kendall/Hunt Publishing, 1992), and Janis Tyler Johnson, *Mothers of Incest Survivors: Another Side of the Story* (Bloomington: Indiana University Press, 1992).

45 In fact, so ready have I been . . . : Susan Suleiman, in an essay entitled "On Maternal Splitting: A Propos of Mary Gordon's *Men and Angels,*" *Signs* 14(1): 25–41 (1988), uses the phrase "ultimate responsibility." She writes, ". . .

what the young child perceives as maternal omnipotence, the mother perceives as absolute or ultimate responsibility. The two perceptions are symmetrical and both are fantasies, for in reality the mother is neither all-powerful in relation to the child nor absolutely responsible for the child's fate," 31.

52   Having a kind of cancer . . . : See Susan M. Love and Karen Lindsey, *Dr. Susan Love's Breast Book* (Reading, MA: Addison-Wesley, 1990) for a comprehensive discussion of the breast, breast cancer, and treatment.

58   Life never worked that way . . . : Women have always worked outside their homes and their labor in the home is productive, but not societally recognized as such. See Elizabeth Fox-Genovese, *Feminism Without Illusions: A Critique of Individualism* (Chapel Hill: University of North Carolina Press, 1991).

59   Susan Suleiman, quoting . . . : Susan Suleiman, "On Maternal Splitting," 39.

Chapter Four

61   Conventional feminine goodness . . . : Mary Field Belenky, Blythe McVicker Clinchy, Nancy Rule Goldberger, and Jill Mattuck Tarule, *Women's Ways of Knowing: The Development of Self, Voice, and Mind* (New York: Basic Books, 1986).

63–64   I have learned . . . : For an extended discussion of the history of the ideas of individualism and their relation to women's history, see Elizabeth Fox-Genovese, *Feminism Without Illusions*. My discussion of these ideas has also profited from reading Edward E. Sampson, "The Deconstruction of the Self," in John Shotter and Kenneth J. Gergen, eds., *Texts of Identity* (London: Sage Publications, 1989); and Linda Kerber, "Some Cautionary Words for Historians," in "Viewpoint: On a Different Voice" in *Signs: Journal of Women in Culture and Society* 11:304–10 (1986).

64   There is nothing permanent . . . : Philip Cushman, "Why the Self Is Empty: Toward a Historically Situated Psychology," *American Psychologist* 45:599–611 (1990).

64   In other words . . . : Edward E. Sampson, "The Deconstruction of the Self," quoting Clifford Geertz, 1.

64   Mothers were to seek . . . : Fox-Genovese, *Feminism Without Illusions*, 125.

65   In the twentieth century . . . : E. Ann Kaplan, "Mothering, Feminism and Representation," 123.

67   Discussing her own book . . . : Carol Gilligan, "Reply" (to critics), in *Signs* 11(2): 326 (1986), and Carol Gilligan, *In a Different Voice: Psychological Theory and Women's Development* (Cambridge, MA: Harvard University Press, 1982).

70   The children's classic . . . : Shel Silverstein, *The Giving Tree* (New York: HarperCollins, 1964).

73   Recent work in social psychology . . . : I have been influenced by two strands of work on subjectivity—one from feminist theory and one from social constructionist theory. Unfortunately, though the two strands are compatible in many ways, there remains a tension that I have found no one able to resolve and which appears in my own writing. If I am saying that voice is social, then

how can I claim that mothers have a subjectivity of their own? For me, the question is unanswerable at this time. Several theoreticians have grappled with this dilemma: the feminist psychoanalyst Jessica Benjamin, in *The Bonds of Love: Psychoanalysis, Feminism, and the Problem of Domination* (New York: Pantheon Books, 1988); Kenneth J. Gergen, in "Feminist Critique of Science and the Challenge of Social Epistemology," in Mary McCanney Gergen, ed., *Feminist Thought and the Structure of Knowledge* (New York: New York University Press, 1988); Rachel T. Hare-Mustin and Jeanne Marecek, "Beyond Difference," in a volume they edited, *Making a Difference: Psychology and the Construction of Gender* (New Haven: Yale University Press, 1990); and John Shotter and Josephine Logan, "The Pervasiveness of Patriarchy: On Finding a Different Voice," in Mary McCanney Gergen, ed., *Feminist Thought and the Structure of Knowledge*.

74   Rather than the self's being . . . : See Kenneth J. Gergen and Mary McCanney Gergen, "Narratives of the Self," in Theodore R. Sarbin and K. E. Scheibe, eds., *Studies in Social Identity* (New York: Praeger, 1983), 265–66; and Harold Goolishian, "The Self: Some Thoughts from a Post-Modernist Perspective on the Intersubjectivity of Mind" (unpublished paper available from the Houston-Galveston Family Therapy Institute, Houston, TX).

74   With this view of the self . . . : For a historical account of the transition between an essential self and a narrative self, see Jerome Bruner, *Acts of Meaning*, and also, Kenneth J. Gergen, *The Saturated Self* (New York: Basic Books, 1991); Louis Sass, "The Self and Its Vicissitudes: An 'Archeological' Study of the Psychoanalytic Avant-Garde," *Social Research* 55:551–607 (1988).

75   A good mother . . . : Restraint on any family member's storytelling has problematic consequences for that individual and for the family as a whole. While much of the clinical literature can be read as documenting the negative effects on children of their parents' inability to accept children's full expression of feelings and thoughts, little attention has been given to the negative effects on parents of restraining their own feelings. I hope that I make clear that sharing is a different activity from burdening. Sharing need not overwhelm children if it respects their developmental and stylistic capacities to listen and respond.

77   Able to conform to . . . : James Agee's *A Death in the Family* (New York: Avon Books, 1957) is one of the most moving accounts I have ever read of a child's view of his mother's grief.

77   It was marvelous . . . : Violet Weingarten, *Intimations of Mortality* (New York: Knopf, 1977).

Chapter Five

85   For unlike us, they . . . : Though statistics vary, those documenting labor force participation rates of women by age of youngest child can be found in Karen A. Matthews and Judith Rodin, "Women's Changing Work Roles: Impact on Health, Family, and Public Policy," *American Psychologist* 44 (11): 1391 (1989). Statistics on females graduating from medical school have been compiled by Cynthia M. Taeuber, ed., *Statistical Handbook on Women in America* (Phoenix, AZ: Oryx Press, 1991).

85   In part, what was unthinkable . . . : For an excellent and readable book

about mothering and careers, see Faye J. Crosby, *Juggling: The Unexpected Advantages of Balancing Career and Home for Women and Their Families* (New York: Free Press, 1991); the guide to further reading in the back of this book is also outstanding.

86   And the bad mother . . . : Immigrant mothers, African-American mothers, and poor mothers are among the mothers who are ill-served by the false dichotomy of family and work. Fathers, too, I argue, are ill served.

86   Psychoanalytic and psychological theories . . . : For a comprehensive review of this literature, see Mary C. Howell, "Effects of Maternal Employment on the Child (II)," *Pediatrics* 52(3):327–43 (1973).

86   Not surprisingly . . . : For a perspective on maternal employment that is consistent with my analysis, see Louise B. Silverstein, "Transforming the Debate about Childcare and Maternal Employment," *American Psychologist* 46(10):1025–32 (1991).

86   "So *immense* are the claims . . .": Quoted from Elaine Showalter, "Women Writers and the Double Standard," in Vivian Gornick and Barbara K. Moran, *Woman in Sexist Society: Studies in Power and Powerlessness* (New York: New American Library, 1972), 446.

87   In two pieces . . . : Violet Brown, "A Working Mother's Job and a Half," *New York Times Magazine,* August 20, 1951, and Violet Brown Weingarten, "Case History of an Ex-Working Mother," *New York Times Magazine,* September 20, 1953.

87   In my mother's first piece . . . : Arlie Hochschild with Anne Machung, *The Second Shift: Working Parents and the Revolution at Home* (New York: Viking and Avon Books, 1989).

96   Since she wants to . . . : See John Bowlby, *Maternal Care and Mental Health* (Geneva: World Health Organization, 1952). For reviews of the literature on the effects on children of maternal employment during the era of the 1950s, see F. Ivan Nye and Lois Wladis Hoffman, *The Employed Mother in America* (New York: Rand McNally, 1963).

96   Knowing what came next . . . : See Pamela Daniels and Kathy Weingarten, *Sooner or Later: The Timing of Parenthood in Adult Lives* (New York: Norton, 1982), chap. 4.

98   On the other hand . . . : For a discussion of medical marriages, see Martha Fowlkes, *Behind Every Successful Man* (New York: Columbia University Press, 1980), and Esther Nitzberg, *Hippocrates' Handmaidens: Women Married to Physicians* (New York: Haworth Press, 1991).

98   The zeitgeist of the times . . . : I knew about Nancy Chodorow's work during its dissertation phase. Her ideas about the importance of shared parenting gave "expert" credibility to the position feminists like me were evolving in consciousness-raising groups. See Nancy Chodorow, *The Reproduction of Mothering: Psychoanalysis and the Sociology of Gender* (Berkeley, CA: University of California Press, 1978). I was also deeply influenced by one of my professors during graduate school, Dr. Mary C. Howell, whose participation in her family life was a model for me. Her research article "Effects of Maternal Employment on the Child (II)" was profoundly reassuring to me, as it would have been to my mother.

100 It mattered immensely to me . . . : The issues surrounding shared or equal parenting are complex. Although I believe that fathers should share parenting, this does not mean that I think it is better to parent with a man than another woman. Nor do I believe that mothers should back off to "let" fathers parent, or that equal parenting will solve the problems of domination that exist. For a discussion of shared parenting and the problem of domination, see Jessica Benjamin, *The Bonds of Love*, 136 and chap. 5; Nancy Chodorow, *The Reproduction of Mothering*; and Diane Ehrensaft, "When Women and Men Mother," in Joyce Trebilcott, ed., *Mothering: Essays in Feminist Theory* (Savage, MD: Rowman & Littlefield, 1983) for complex discussions of these issues.

101 I knew all this . . . : I am sure that a factor in my decision-making was the flexibility I had in scheduling my work. I could earn a full-time salary while doing my work after the children were asleep.

101 In a letter to . . . : The work of the four women in this project, Betty Carter, Peggy Papp, Olga Silverstein, and Marianne Walters, published in *The Invisible Web: Gender Patterns in Family Relationships* (New York: Guilford Press, 1988), was invaluable to me, as was the pioneering work of Rachel T. Hare-Mustin, bringing a feminist analysis squarely into the family-therapy field in "A Feminist Approach to Family Therapy," *Family Process* 17:181–94 (1978).

103 Arlie Hochschild writes . . . : Arlie Hochschild with Anne Machung, *The Second Shift*, 57.

105 This theme expressed . . . : For an excellent discussion of the ways marriage rather than motherhood handicaps women's careers, see Faye J. Crosby, *Juggling*.

107 I will also ask . . . : Sandra Scarr, Deborah Phillips, and Kathleen McCartney, "Working Mothers and Their Families," *American Psychologist* 44 (11): 1405 (1989).

108 Pleck offers another . . . : Joseph Pleck, *Working Wives/Working Husbands* (Newbury Park, CA: Sage, 1985), 93.

Chapter Six

111 Long before I had ever heard . . . : My mother was referring to the play *A Doll's House* by Henrik Ibsen (New York: S. French, 1972).

112 Yet it is dominance . . . : Philip W. Blumstein and Pepper Schwartz make the point in *American Couples: Money, Work, Sex* (New York: Morrow, 1983), 318–30, that men have a need for dominance but there is no corresponding need for submission in women. Indeed, women are reluctant to dominate. For a powerful story about dominance and submission in marriage and the alternative of mutuality, see Zora Neale Hurston, *Their Eyes Were Watching God* (New York: Harper & Row, 1990), first published in 1937.

113 Reflecting on my thoughts and feelings . . . : Miriam M. Johnson, *Strong Mothers, Weak Wives* (Berkeley, CA: University of California Press, 1988).

113 She disagrees . . . : See Dorothy Dinnerstein, *The Mermaid and the Minotaur: Sexual Arrangements and Human Malaise* (New York: Harper & Row,

1976), and Nancy Chodorow, *The Reproduction of Mothering: Psychoanalysis and the Sociology of Gender.*

113 She urges us to note . . . : Miriam M. Johnson, *Strong Mothers, Weak Wives,* 9.

113 In recent years . . . : See, for example, Kerrie James and Laurie Mac-Kinnon, "The Incestuous Family Revisited: A Critical Analysis of Family Therapy Myths," *Journal of Marital and Family Therapy* 16 (1): 72–88 (1990), and Louise DeSalvo, *Virginia Woolf: The Impact of Childhood Sexual Abuse on Her Life and Work* (New York: Ballantine Books, 1989).

114 I know from personal . . . : I wish to make it perfectly clear that dominance in any form, by males or females, is harmful to the recipients. That it is harmful to the perpetrators is also the case, but our understanding of this must not interfere with our willingness to hold perpetrators responsible for their acts. As we learn about their lives, we may feel compassion for their situations, yet we must insist on remorse and change.

116 When I read . . . : Nina Schneider, *The Woman Who Lived in a Prologue* (New York: Avon Books, 1979).

116 My first-born . . . : Ibid., 158–59.

118 Mothers who do fear violence . . . : It is not my purpose here to advocate that women defend themselves against their male partners. As of this writing, researchers concerned with domestic violence are debating whether a woman places herself at more or less risk if she expresses anger or fights back. For contrasting statements, see Judith Lewis Herman, *Trauma and Recovery* (New York: Basic Books, 1992), 75, and Angela Browne and Kirk R. Williams, "Are Women as Violent as Men?: Research on 'Domestic Violence' and Considerations for the Field" (available from the first author, University of Massachusetts, Department of Psychiatry, 55 Lake Avenue North, Worcester, MA 02115), 22.

118 This moment, brief though it may be . . . : See Lenore Walker, *The Battered Woman* (New York: Harper & Row, 1979), and Judith Lewis Herman, *Trauma and Recovery,* chap. 4.

118 Children who witness . . . : Robert S. Pynoos and Spencer Eth, "Children Traumatized by Witnessing Acts of Personal Violence: Homicide, Rape, or Suicide Behavior," in Spencer Eth and Robert S. Pynoos, eds., *Posttraumatic Stress Disorder in Children* (Washington, D.C.: American Psychiatric Press, 1985).

122 There is little doubt . . . : See Lenore Walker, *The Battered Woman,* 76.; Judith Lewis Herman, *Trauma and Recovery,* chap. 4; and Robert S. Pynoos and Spencer Eth, "Children Traumatized by Witnessing Acts of Personal Violence."

123 I wanted to know . . . : See Jessica Benjamin, *The Bonds of Love: Psychoanalysis, Feminism, and the Problem of Domination.*

124 According to this view . . . : Miriam M. Johnson, *Strong Mothers, Weak Wives,* 161.

125 Johnson's theory . . . : Ibid.

125 The apparent contradiction . . . : Ibid.

127   As I have mentioned . . . : See Judith Lewis Herman, *Trauma and Recovery*, 34.

127   Wife battering and rape . . . : See Lenore Walker, *The Battered Woman*.

128   She was affected . . . : The issue of the effects of violence on children over time is a critical area for research. Several good sources in exploring this topic are: Robert S. Pynoos and Spencer Eth, "Children Traumatized by Witnessing Acts of Personal Violence"; Beverly Rivera and Cathy Spatz Widom, "Childhood Victimization and Violent Offending," *Violence and Victims* 5:(1):19–35 (1990); and Gail Ryan, "Victim to Victimizer: Rethinking Victim Treatment," *Journal of Interpersonal Violence* 4(3):325–41 (1989). Differences in effects can be attributed to both characteristics of the violent event—for instance, context, severity, and chronicity—and characteristics of the child witness, such as gender, age, and race.

132   Part of what drives . . . : In this anecdote, as in many others in this book, I have selected events that may be outside the usual definitions people use to categorize an episode as abusive or not for the purpose of showing that meaning cannot be interpreted solely from external characteristics, but inheres in subjective appraisal of experience. This haircut was traumatic for me, and I believe that the intergenerational family dynamics that surround this circumstance can be understood from a trauma perspective. At the same time, I hope that my emphasis on dominance makes clear that I do not believe that the intergenerational transmission of abuse can be understood without a gender analysis, in this case one that focuses on male dominance. See Judith Lewis Herman, "Considering Sex Offenders: A Model of Addiction," in *Signs: Journal of Women in Culture and Society* 13(4): 695–724 (1988). I could have described the intergenerational transmission process of abuse through an example of physical, emotional, or sexual abuse, but these descriptions are relatively more common. My point is precisely to alert people to the more subtle locations in which abuse and violation, dominance and submission patterns exist and evolve. It is not my intention to compare the deleterious effects of a haircut with those of, for example, rape. For a discussion of the intergenerational patterns surrounding abuse, see the work of Denise Gelinas, for example, "The Persisting Negative Effects of Incest," *Psychiatry* 46:312–32 (1983).

132   In fact, studies have shown . . . : See Angela Browne, for the Council on Scientific Affairs, "Violence Against Women: Relevance for Medical Practitioners," *Journal of the American Medical Association* 267 (23): 3186–87 (June 17, 1992).

132   Susan Moller Okin, a political scientist . . . : Susan Moller Okin, *Justice, Gender, and the Family* (New York: Basic Books, 1989). In one section of the book she draws on the work of Alfred O. Hirschman, 136–38.

133   Nor did I ever worry . . . : See Angela Browne, "The Victim's Experience: Pathways to Disclosure," *Psychotherapy* 28(1):150–56 (1991).

133   They are rendered . . . : Susan Moller Okin, *Justice, Gender, and the Family*, 138–39.

134   Most commonly, divorce for women . . . : Lenore J. Weitzman, in *The Divorce Revolution: The Unexpected Consequences for Women and Children in*

America (New York: Free Press, 1985), cites a 73% decline in income, whereas Greg J. Duncan and Saul D. Hoffman, in "A Reconsideration of the Economic Consequences of Marital Dissolution," *Demography* 25 (4): 641 (1988), cite the lower figure, 33%, which they believe is temporary. See also Susan Faludi, *Backlash: The Undeclared War Against American Women* (New York: Crown, 1991), for a discussion of this controversy.

134 In *Mothers on Trial* . . . : Phyllis Chesler, *Mothers on Trial: The Battle for Children and Custody* (New York: McGraw-Hill, 1986).

135 One consequence of some modern divorces . . . : See Sue Miller's *The Good Mother* (New York: Harper & Row, 1986) for a provocative fictional account of contemporary custody issues.

135 Husbands sue mothers for custody . . . : Phyllis Chesler, *Mothers on Trial*, xi.

135 In a moving personal story . . . : The name plays on associations to Anna Karenina and the Greek goddess Demeter, who loses her daughter.

135 "I thought I had to make . . .": Anna Demeter, *Legal Kidnaping* (Boston: Beacon Press, 1977), 1.

136 One of Anna's children . . . : Anna Demeter, *Legal Kidnaping*, 125.

137 For heterosexual couples, however . . . : See Dorothy Dinnerstein, *The Mermaid and the Minotaur*, and Nancy Chodorow, *The Reproduction of Mothering*.

137–38 In a recent "Hers" column . . . : See Patricia Raybon, "Stolen Promises," *New York Times Magazine*, May 3, 1992.

Chapter Seven

142 "the cultural elites . . .": the *Boston Globe*, 11 June 1992, 1.

142 As Stacey writes . . . : Judith Stacey, *Brave New Families: Stories of Domestic Upheaval in Late Twentieth Century America* (New York: Basic Books, 1990), 252.

143 Implicit in these tales . . . : See Phoebe Kazdin Schnitzer, "Tales of the Absent Father: Applying the 'Story' Metaphor in Family Therapy," *Family Process* 32(4):441–58 (1993), for a discussion of how maternal storytelling influences a child's experience of his absent father.

143 First, they suggest . . . : See Mona Simpson, *The Lost Father* (New York: Knopf, 1992).

143 I find the subtext of blaming . . . : Family therapist Lynn Hoffman puts this point most succinctly in her teaching. Elaborations of it can be found in Luigi Boscolo, Gianfranco Cecchin, Lynn Hoffman, and Peggy Penn, *Milan Systemic Family Therapy* (New York: Basic Books, 1987).

144 My mother not only kept . . . : See Phoebe Kazdin Schnitzer, "Tales of the Absent Father," for a discussion of how maternal storytelling influences a child's experience of his absent father.

146 Although the mental-health community . . . : See Louise B. Silverstein, "Transforming the Debate about Child Care and Maternal Employment," *American Psychologist* 46(10):1030 (1991).

147 One representation . . . : Vicky Phares, "Where's Poppa? The Relative Lack of Attention to the Role of Fathers in Child and Adolescent Psychopathol-

ogy," *American Psychologist* 47(5):656–64 (1992); S. T. Boyd, "Study of the Father: Research Methods," *American Behavioral Scientist* 29:112–28 (1985).

147 Prior to the 1970s . . . : Phyllis Bronstein and Carolyn Pape Cowan, eds., *Fatherhood Today: Men's Changing Role in the Family* (New York: Wiley, 1988), 6.

147 Newer studies show . . . : See Michael E. Lamb, ed., *The Role of the Father in Child Development* (New York: Wiley, 1986), and Phyllis Bronstein and Carolyn Pape Cowan, eds., *Fatherhood Today*.

147 In some studies . . . : See John Lewis McAdoo, "Changing Perspectives on the Role of the Black Father," in Phyllis Bronstein and Carolyn Pape Cowan, eds., *Fatherhood Today,* 82; and E. Mavis Hetherington, "Coping with Family Transitions: Winners, Losers, and Survivors," *Child Development* 60:1–114 (1989).

147 But this indirect presence . . . : Ibid.

147 One study, however . . . : Andrew J. Cherlin, Frank F. Furstenberg, Jr., P. Lindsay Chase-Lansdale, Kathleen E. Kiernan, Philip K. Robins, Donna Ruane Morrison, Julien O. Teitler, "Longitudinal Studies of Effects of Divorce on Children in Great Britain and the United States," *Science* 252:1386–89 (June 7, 1991).

147 They concluded that the effect . . . : Ibid., 1388. Another aspect of father absence in relation to divorce is discussed by Frank F. Furstenberg, Jr., and Andrew Cherlin in *Divided Families: What Happens to Children When Parents Part* (Cambridge, MA: Harvard University Press, 1991). The authors note that for many men, marriage and parenthood are a package deal; "their ties to their children, and their feelings of responsibility for their children, depend on their ties to their wives," 118. Moreover, many men have trouble dealing with their children without assistance from their wives. Psychologist and family therapist Ronald F. Levant teaches fathers parenting skills. See Ronald F. Levant and John Kelly, *Between Father and Child* (New York: Penguin, 1991). For a more academic presentation of their ideas, see Ronald F. Levant, "Education for Fatherhood," in Phyllis Bronstein and Carolyn Pape Cowan, eds., *Fatherhood Today,* 253–75.

149 This interpretation is supported . . . : The findings in this paragraph are reported in Murray A. Strauss and Richard J. Gelles, "How Violent Are American Families? Estimates from the National Family Violence Resurvey and Other Studies," in Murray A. Strauss and Richard J. Gelles, *Physical Violence in American Families: Risk Factors and Adaptations to Violence in 8,145 Families* (New Brunswick, NJ: Transaction Publishers, 1990), and Angela Browne and Kirk R. Williams, "Are Women as Violent as Men?"

149 Mothers observe firsthand . . . : Gerald T. Hotaling and David B. Sugarman, "An Analysis of Risk Markers in Husband to Wife Violence: The Current State of Knowledge," *Violence and Victims* 1(2):101–24 (1986).

149 The mother was . . . : Lenore Walker, *The Battered Woman.*

150 It reminds me . . . : Dante Cicchetti, "Developmental Consequences of Child Maltreatment," paper presented at the Harvard Medical School Conference on Psychological Trauma, Boston, May 29–30, 1992.

150   Securely attached children . . . : Dante Cicchetti, "Developmental Consequences of Child Maltreatment."

151   According to sociologist Christopher Jencks . . . : Christopher Jencks, *Rethinking Social Policy: Race, Poverty, and the Underclass* (Cambridge, MA: Harvard University Press, 1992), 32. See also Andrew Billingsley, *Black Families in White America* (Englewood Cliffs, NJ: Prentice Hall, 1968), for an in-depth description of different black extended-family types and their positioning within mainstream white American society.

151   Also, since many unmarried . . . : Christopher Jencks, *Rethinking Social Policy*, 32.

151   Although families with children . . . : In 1988, 7% of families with children headed by a married couple were poor in contrast to 45% headed by a mother alone. This fact is cited in Frank F. Furstenberg, Jr., and Andrew Cherlin, *Divided Families*, 45.

152   Lesbians are no longer . . . : Sally Crawford, "Lesbian Families: Psychosocial Stress and the Family-building Process," in Boston Lesbian Psychologies Collective, ed., *Lesbian Psychologies: Explorations and Challenges* (Urbana: University of Illinois, 1987), 195.

152   For lesbians, the two identities . . . : Nancy Polikoff, "Lesbians Choosing Children: The Personal Is Political Revisited," in Sandra Pollack and Jeanne Vaughn, eds., *Politics of the Heart: A Lesbian Anthology* (Ithaca, NY: Firebrand Books, 1987), 49.

152   As Laura Benkov points out . . . : Laura Benkov, *Reinventing the Family: The Emerging Story of Lesbian and Gay Parents* (New York: Crown, in press).

153   Benkov cites the figure . . . : Laura Benkov, *Lesbian Parenting: Redefining the Family*, 1994. A dissertation submitted to the Graduate Faculty in Psychology, The City University of New York, 1990, 51.

154   Second, never-married mothers . . . : Harriette Pipes McAdoo, "Changes in the Formation and Structure of Black Families: The Impact on Black Women," *Working Paper No. 182* (Wellesley, MA: Wellesley College Center for Research on Women, 1988), 12.

154   African-American families are not . . . : See Carol B. Stack, *All Our Kin: Strategies for Survival in a Black Community* (New York: Harper & Row, 1974), and Nancy Boyd-Franklin, *Black Families in Therapy: A Multisystems Approach* (New York: Guilford Press, 1989).

155   In Perri Klass's novel . . . : Perri Klass, *Other Women's Children* (New York: Random House, 1990).

156   In *Iron John: A Book about Men* . . . : Robert Bly, *Iron John: A Book about Men* (Reading, MA: Addison-Wesley, 1990), 92.

156   Bly asserts that men . . . : Robert Bly, *Iron John*.

157   In the Iron John World . . . : Karen A. Matthews and Judith Rodin, "Women's Changing Work Roles," 1389.

157   In 1986, 54% of mothers . . . : Louise B. Silverstein, "Transforming the Debate about Child Care and Maternal Employment," 1025.

157   Currently, the unequal sharing . . . : Arlie Hochschild with Anne Machung, *The Second Shift*.

157 Though estimates of time spent . . . : Adele Eskeles Gottfried and Allen W. Gottfried, *Maternal Employment and Children's Development* (New York: Plenum Press, 1988).

157 In her book . . . : Faye J. Crosby, *Juggling*, 151.

159 Walking into his son's room . . . : Paul Monette, *Borrowed Time: An AIDS Memoir* (New York: Avon Books, 1988), 341.

161 Deborah Tannen, in her book . . . : Deborah Tannen, *You Just Don't Understand: Women and Men in Conversation* (New York: Morrow, 1990).

Chapter Eight

167 It is written in many places . . . : See Carol Gilligan, *In a Different Voice;* Harriet Goldhor Lerner, *The Dance of Intimacy* (New York: Harper & Row, 1989); Letty Cottin Pogrebin, *Among Friends: Who We Like, Why We Like Them, and What We Do with Them* (New York: McGraw-Hill, 1987); and Lillian B. Rubin, *Intimate Strangers: Men and Women Together* (New York: Harper & Row, 1983).

167 According to this story . . . : Adrienne Rich, *Of Woman Born*, Tenth Anniversary Ed. (New York: Norton, 1986), 226.

167 I don't know how recent . . . : Psychoanalytic object-relations theory is the psychoanalytic theory that underlies Nancy Chodorow's work, a prime exponent of this point of view; see her *The Reproduction of Mothering.*

168 Chodorow also believes . . . : Ibid., 110.

170 Is this the moment . . . : Carol Gilligan's discussion of a boy's "relational crisis" in early childhood is consistent with the ideas I have put forward here. See Carol Gilligan, "Women's Psychological Development: Implications for Psychotherapy," in Carol Gilligan, Annie G. Rogers, and Deborah L. Tolman, *Women, Girls, & Psychotherapy: Reframing Resistance* (Binghampton, NY: Harrington Park Press, 1991).

171 Blaming older men . . . : Robert Bly, *Iron John*, 19.

173 Studies of men . . . : See Angela Browne and Kirk R. Williams, "Gender, Intimacy, and Lethal Violence: Trends from 1976–1987," *Gender and Society* 7(1):78–98 (1993).

177 Though the gender story . . . : Lyman C. Wynne, "The Epigenesis of Relational Systems: A Model for Understanding Family Development," *Family Process* 23:297–318 (1984).

179 It sometimes happens . . . : Z. D. Gurevitch, "The Power of Not Understanding: The Meeting of Conflicting Identities," *The Journal of Applied Behavioral Science* 25:161–73 (1989), 161.

Chapter Nine

188 Like a person . . . : See Judith Lewis Herman, *Trauma and Recovery*, 35.

190 As a clinician in training . . . : See John Bowlby, *Attachment and Loss*, Vol. 1, *Attachment* (New York: Basic Books, 1969), and *Attachment and Loss*, Vol. 2, *Separation* (New York: Basic Books, 1973); Margaret S. Mahler, *On Human Symbiosis and the Vicissitudes of Individuation* (New York: International Universities Press, 1968); and Margaret S. Mahler, Fred Pine, and Anni

Bergman, *The Psychological Birth of the Human Infant: Symbiosis and Individuation* (New York: Basic Books, 1975).

190   Curiously, they have formed . . . : For a detailed account of early separation theories, see Jessica Benjamin, *The Bonds of Love.*

190   One of the theories I learned . . . : Ibid.

190   In contrast, the other theory . . . : Margaret S. Mahler, Fred Pine, and Anni Bergman, *The Psychological Birth of the Human Infant.*

190   The first theory lays the foundations . . . : John Bowlby's work is part of the object-relations school of psychoanalysis.

190   Whereas both perspectives . . . : See Carol Gilligan, *In a Different Voice;* Carol Gilligan, Annie G. Rogers, and Deborah L. Tolman, *Women, Girls, & Psychotherapy;* Harold D. Grotevant and Catherine R. Cooper, eds., *Adolescent Development in the Family: New Directions for Child Development* (San Francisco: Jossey-Bass, 1983); Susan J. Frank, Catherine Butler Avery, and Mark S. Laman, "Young Adults' Perceptions of Their Relationships with Their Parents: Individual Differences in Connectedness, Competence, and Emotional Autonomy," *Developmental Psychology* 24(5): 729–37 (1988).

191   By omitting the parents from theorizing . . . : See Pamela Daniels and Kathy Weingarten, *Sooner or Later: The Timing of Parenthood in Adult Lives* (New York: Norton, 1982). In this book, parental development is assumed, and one focus is on the ways children influence parental development.

191   Where traditional theories . . . : I have been influenced by the work of Jessica Benjamin, who has theorized that "mutual recognition" is as significant a developmental goal as separation from the beginning of infant development. Extrapolating her thinking to adolescence, I think "mutual knowing" may constitute "separation" at this stage. Benjamin, writing about infancy, says that "the issue is not how we become free of the other, but how we actively engage and make ourselves known in relationship to the other"; see Jessica Benjamin, *Bonds of Love,* 18. I think this notion has applicability for adolescence as well. In Stuart T. Hauser with Sally I. Powers and Gil G. Noam, *Adolescents and Their Families: Paths of Ego Development* (New York: Free Press, 1991), there is a perspective on adolescence that is compatible with the ideas I am presenting here.

191   Adolescence has been called . . . : Peter Blos, *On Adolescence: A Psychoanalytic Interpretation* (New York: Free Press, 1962), 12.

192   In the contemporary story line . . . : Robert Bly, *Iron John,* 19.

192   Mothers, he says . . . : Ibid., 12.

193   In the story . . . : Ibid., 258.

200   They had great passions . . . : See Marianne Hirsch, *The Mother-Daughter Plot,* 170–71, for a discussion of anger in the mother-daughter relationship.

200   "The birth of dialogue" . . . : Z. D. Gurevitch, "The Other Side of Dialogue: On Making the Other Strange and the Experience of Otherness," *American Journal of Sociology* 93(5): 1189 (1988).

201   Carol Gilligan and her colleagues . . . : Lyn Mikel Brown and Carol Gilligan, "The Psychology of Women and the Development of Girls," paper

presented at the Laurel-Harvard Conference on the Psychology of Girls, Cleveland, Ohio, April 1990, 38.

201 When my son Ben . . . : Feenie Ziner, *Within This Wilderness: The True Story of a Mother's Journey to Rediscover Her Son* (New York: Norton, 1978).

202 " '. . . I just don't understand . . .": Feenie Ziner, *Within This Wilderness*, 114.

202 "three rough, ax-hewn steps . . .": Ibid., 224–25.

205 African-American women . . . : See, for example, Alice Walker, *In Search of Our Mothers' Gardens* (New York: Harcourt Brace Jovanovich, 1983), and Sarah Lawrence Lightfoot, *Balm in Gilead: Journey of a Healer* (Reading, MA: Addison-Wesley, 1988).

205 Whether any mother and daughter . . . : See Teri Apter, *Altered Loves: Mothers and Daughters During Adolescence* (New York: St. Martins, 1990), for a description of adolescent separation issues that is consistent with the framework presented here.

Chapter Ten

210 As Sara Ruddick has said . . . : Sara Ruddick, *Maternal Thinking*, 40.

210 Families can also be the place . . . : Edward E. Sampson, "The Deconstruction of the Self," in John Shotter and Kenneth J. Gergen, eds., *Texts of Identity*, 1–19.

211 We must try to decode meaning . . . : Although I focus on spoken language, I believe that meaning is communicated through symbols and gestures, and that they, too, can be understood and resisted.

212 But the experience of cancer . . . : See Arthur Kleinman, *The Illness Narratives: Suffering, Healing and the Human Condition* (New York: Basic Books, 1988).

213 I support wholeheartedly . . . : See *Ms. Magazine*, May/June 1993, for an extended discussion of the politics of breast cancer.

ACKNOWLEDGMENTS

I really wanted to write this book. For also wanting me to write it, and for understanding that I would need to write about them, I am grateful to my children and my husband—Ben, Miranda, and Hilary Worthen—and to my sister and my father, Jan Greenberg and Victor Weingarten. All five have supported my writing in the most generous and precious way, by not asking that their views of or feelings about my material be considered.

Many people have encouraged me, supported me, listened to me, and taken care of me during the many phases of my life that have run concurrently with the writing of this book. To Ruth Balser, Carol Becker, Laura Benkov, Michele Bograd, Sara Cobb, Risa Delong, Abigail Erdmann, Chris Gilman, Jan Greenberg, Judith Kates, William Kates, Joan Labby, Kathy Lancaster, Debra Lang, Monica Meehan McNamara, Lois Natchez, Joan Oleson, Peggy Penn, Megan Purvee, Sallyann Roth, Susan Siroty, Jennifer Slack, Joan Stein, Carter Umbarger, Linda Weingarten, Mollie Weingarten, Victor Weingarten, Eleanor Worthen, Helena Worthen, Hilary Worthen, Mark Worthen, and Regina Yando I acknowledge the profound difference attentive love can make.

Many colleagues have made a difference. At Judge Baker Children's Center in Boston, the members of my family-therapy supervisors' group, with whom I have been meeting since 1980, have known how to move flexibly between colleagueship, friendship, and family. Members of the Clinical Service Program, especially Glenda Alderman, Holly Bishop, and Christina Crowe, have also been supportive and caring. Amy Nevis and Gerry Koocher made it clear during my illness that, both officially and personally, they wanted to be accommodating. This has meant a great deal to me. My colleagues at the Family Institute of Cambridge have welcomed me to speak with all the intensity I can muster about my cancer experiences. I am enormously grateful that I work with people who want to know me.

I have been fortunate to have wonderful doctors, nurses, social workers, and health workers, who are competent, caring people, and who have been willing to have intimate interactions with me. I wish to thank Mark Aronson, Richard Chasin, Jay Harris, Hester Hill, Richard Kahn, Sam Kaplan, Frances Kiel, Clinton Koufman, Susan LaViolette, Richard Pasternak, Victoria Pittman, Marcie Richardson, Lowell Schnipper, Faye Snider, and Jacqueline Tschetter for their attentive care. Without their expertise, I wouldn't be here; without their conversation, this book wouldn't be.

Several people read earlier drafts of selected chapters and encouraged me in my writing. I thank Rosalind Barnett, Laura Benkov, Abigail Erdmann, Carol Gilligan, Ronald F. Levant, Jade McGleughlin, Monica McGoldrick, Susan Bangs Munro, and Sallyann Roth. Others have read earlier drafts of the full manuscript and patiently steadied me when I lost confidence: Carol Becker, Sara Cobb, Risa Delong, Jan Greenberg, Margaret Holt, Kathleen Lancaster, Lois Natchez, Peggy Penn, Victor Weingarten, Eleanor Worthen, Helena Worthen, Hilary Worthen, and Mark Worthen.

Carol Becker, Laura Benkov, Lois Natchez, and Hilary Worthen have been loving companions throughout the entire process. Jo Ann Miller worked with me to transform the initial rambling manuscript into a work with a single unifying frame. Her generosity and intelligence were essential to this book. Jessica Daniel and Sara Ruddick gave me their professional opinions about the final draft. The book is better for their readings; the remaining problems fall squarely on my plate. My mother-in-law, Eleanor Worthen, has read multiple drafts of this book, writing me wonderfully useful notes along the margins of the pages. I have often felt her skill and faith as a palpable presence beside me as I write.

Though very few of my clients' stories appear in these pages— slightly altered and disguised, at that—I feel enormous gratitude for the many hours I have spent with them as we patiently become intimate with each other. I cannot adequately express how significant to my own growth sharing their lives has been.

My agent, Lynn Nesbit, determinedly traveled this book's journey with me, connecting me to my editor, Pat Strachan. Sometimes my pleasure in working with Pat makes me weep at my good fortune. Her intelligence, grace, and compassion have been the sweetest gift.

Finally, the work of many writers whose names do not hold a central place in this book have significantly influenced it. I wish to acknowledge my gratitude to: Laura Benkov, Mary M. Gergen, Rachel T. Hare-Mustin, Carolyn Heilbrun, Marianne Hirsch, Audre Lorde, Adrienne Rich, Sara Ruddick, Violet Weingarten, and the members of the Women's Project in Family Therapy.